AF771649

Thieme

Neurosurgery Infographics

Nitin Agarwal, MD
Associate Professor, Neurological Surgery and Bioengineering
Director, Minimally Invasive Spine and Robotics Surgery
Director, Complex and Minimally Invasive Spine Deformity Fellowship
Director, Spine Computational Outcomes Learning Institute
Department of Neurological Surgery
University of Pittsburgh School of Medicine
Pittsburgh, Pennsylvania, USA.

David T. Fernandes Cabral, MD
Assistant Professor of Neurological Surgery
Director of Resident Education
Department of Neurological Surgery
University of Pittsburgh School of Medicine
University of Pittsburgh Medical Center
Pittsburgh, Pennsylvania, USA

277 illustrations

Thieme
New York • Stuttgart • Delhi • Rio de Janeiro

Library of Congress Cataloging-in-Publication Data is available from the publisher.

Thieme Medical Publishers, Inc.
333 Seventh Avenue, 18th Floor,
New York, NY 10001, USA
www.thieme.com
+1 800 782 3488,
customerservice@thieme.com

Cover design: © Thieme
Cover image source: Illustration created by Carol Hrejsa/ © Thieme
Typesetting by TNQ Tech Private Limited, India

Printed in India by Replika Press Pvt. Ltd. 5 4 3 2

DOI: 10.1055/b000001078

ISBN: 978-1-68420-767-1

Also available as eBook:
eISBN (PDF): 978-1-68420-682-7
eISBN (epub): 978-1-68420-683-4

Important note: Medicine is an ever-changing science undergoing continual development. Research and clinical experience are continually expanding our knowledge, in particular our knowledge of proper treatment and drug therapy. Insofar as this book mentions any dosage or application, readers may rest assured that the authors, editors, and publishers have made every effort to ensure that such references are in accordance with **the state of knowledge at the time of production of the book.**

Nevertheless, this does not involve, imply, or express any guarantee or responsibility on the part of the publishers in respect to any dosage instructions and forms of applications stated in the book. **Every user is requested to examine carefully** the manufacturers' leaflets accompanying each drug and to check, if necessary in consultation with a physician or specialist, whether the dosage schedules mentioned therein or the contraindications stated by the manufacturers differ from the statements made in the present book. Such examination is particularly important with drugs that are either rarely used or have been newly released on the market. Every dosage schedule or every form of application used is entirely at the user's own risk and responsibility. The authors and publishers request every user to report to the publishers any discrepancies or inaccuracies noticed. If errors in this work are found after publication, errata will be posted at www.thieme. com on the product description page.

Some of the product names, patents, and registered designs referred to in this book are in fact registered trademarks or proprietary names even though specific reference to this fact is not always made in the text. Therefore, the appearance of a name without designation as proprietary is not to be construed as a representation by the publisher that it is in the public domain.

Thieme addresses people of all gender identities equally. We encourage our authors to use gender-neutral or gender-equal expressions wherever the context allows.

MIX
Paper | Supporting responsible forestry
FSC www.fsc.org FSC™ C016779

To my family for their unconditional support.

To my patients for teaching me on a daily basis.

To my colleagues for helping me carry the message.

To my mentors for educating me in the art of neurosurgery.

Nitin Agarwal, MD

To my beloved wife, Varuna, whose unwavering love, patience, and quiet strength have sustained me through countless late nights and long years of study, writing, and practice. Thank you for keeping our home a true haven and for believing in me even when the path felt uncertain.

To my mother, Betty, and my late father, Basilio, whose foundational love, sacrifices, and encouragement shaped who I am today; I carry your support with me always.

And to my brother, Daniel, thank you for your constant trust in me, for championing my professional dreams from the very start.

David T. Fernandes Cabral, MD

Contents

Videos

Foreword

Neurosurgery Infographics is exactly the kind of resource our field needs right now. As the volume and complexity of neurosurgical knowledge continue to grow, we need learning tools that meet trainees and clinicians where they are—tools that are rigorous without being inaccessible. Drs. Nitin Agarwal and David T. Fernandes Cabral have done precisely that.

What sets this book apart is how well it balances breadth and clarity. The visual abstracts and concise summaries cover the full scope of our specialty without sacrificing depth. The peer-reviewed infographics provide clarity without oversimplifying—they give readers a solid grasp of core principles while inviting deeper exploration. That is a genuinely difficult balance to strike, and they have struck it well.

I can see this book being useful across the full spectrum of training and practice. For medical students heading into sub-internships, it builds confidence and clinical context. For residents managing packed schedules, it is an efficient way to reinforce what matters. And for practicing neurosurgeons, it offers a quick, reliable refresher. The visual format works—it improves retention and supports real clinical application.

Most importantly, *Neurosurgery Infographics* reflects something I care deeply about: the responsibility we share to teach well and to keep innovating in how we do it. Education is not static, and neither is neurosurgery. This book embraces that—and will serve our trainees for years to come.

I recommend this book wholeheartedly. May it spark curiosity, sharpen understanding, and strengthen the educational foundation of our next generation of neurosurgeons. In a field where change is the only constant, *Neurosurgery Infographics* is a timely and welcome contribution.

Martina A. Stippler, MD
President, Congress of Neurological Surgeons
Schaumburg, Illinois, USA

Preface

Neurosurgery is a field of profound complexity, an interplay of anatomy, pathology, technology, and human experience. Yet at its core lies a simple truth: to treat the nervous system effectively, one must understand clearly. That clarity is what inspired *Neurosurgery Infographics*.

When Nitin Agarwal and I began this project, our goal was straightforward yet ambitious: to distill the vast, intricate truths of cranial, spinal, and peripheral nerve surgery into visuals that speak at a glance, and then invite deeper study. We envisioned a resource that spares the learner from getting lost in text-dense atlases or sprawling monographs and instead offers high-impact infographics: each one a stop-light moment of insight.

We targeted the junior resident waking at dawn for rounds, the medical student striving to orient themselves in their neurosurgery rotation, and the advanced practice provider seeking a rapid review. For each, we wanted: clarity, immediacy, fidelity to evidence, and elegance of presentation. Consequently, this book presents one hundred peer-reviewed visual summaries, each crafted to anchor key neurosurgical disorders with precision and accessibility.

Of course, simplicity does not mean superficiality. Behind every infographic lies rigorous scholarship, curated by our contributors and vetted through review. We embraced rather than eliminated complexity; but offered it in a different form: sculpted into graphic form, layered for review, and designed to prompt memory, comprehension, and application.

Whether you are encountering a subdural hematoma in the emergency department, navigating lumbar degenerative stenosis in clinic, or reviewing nerve entrapment syndromes on the ward, this guide is meant to be your companion. Flip open a page. Let the anatomy, the algorithm, the imaging, the decision-tree speak. Then dive deeper into the narrative when needed.

In writing this preface, we reflect on the many mentors, patients, and peers who have shaped my understanding of neurosurgery, and whose questions inspired this work. To learners everywhere, we offer this volume as a bridge: from uncertainty to informed action, from novice to confident reviewer.

May this guide serve you well in the hours before the first case, the moments between the rounds and the OR, and the lifelong journey of surgical mastery.

David T. Fernandes Cabral, MD
Assistant Professor of Neurological Surgery
Director of Resident Education
Department of Neurological Surgery
University of Pittsburgh School of Medicine
University of Pittsburgh Medical Center
Pittsburgh, Pennsylvania, USA

Acknowledgments

We extend our deepest gratitude to Regan Shanahan and Samuel Adida, two stellar medical students from the University of Pittsburgh School of Medicine whose tireless effort, dedication, and attention to detail were instrumental in bringing this book to life. Their commitment and their willingness to go above and beyond made an immeasurable difference in the quality and completeness of this work. Nitin and I are profoundly grateful for their partnership, and we take great pride in knowing that the future of neurosurgery will be shaped by individuals as capable, thoughtful, and inspiring as Regan and Samuel.

David T. Fernandes Cabral, MD
Assistant Professor of Neurological Surgery
Director of Resident Education
Department of Neurological Surgery
University of Pittsburgh School of Medicine
University of Pittsburgh Medical Center
Pittsburgh, Pennsylvania, USA

Contributors

Nitin Agarwal, MD
Associate Professor of Neurological Surgery and Bioengineering
Director, Minimally Invasive Spine and Robotics Surgery
Director, Complex and Minimally Invasive Spine Deformity Fellowship
Director, Spine Computational Outcomes Learning Institute
Department of Neurological Surgery
University of Pittsburgh School of Medicine
Pittsburgh, Pennsylvania, USA

David T. Fernandes Cabral, MD
Assistant Professor of Neurological Surgery
Director of Resident Education
Department of Neurological Surgery
University of Pittsburgh School of Medicine
University of Pittsburgh Medical Center
Pittsburgh, Pennsylvania, USA

Samuel Adida, MS
Medical Student
Department of Neurological Surgery
University of Pittsburgh School of Medicine
Pittsburgh, Pennsylvania, USA

Regan Shanahan, MS
Medical Student
Department of Neurological Surgery
University of Pittsburgh School of Medicine
Pittsburgh, Pennsylvania, USA

Reviewers

Alexander I. Evins, MD
Assistant Professor of Neurological Surgery and
Neurosurgical Innovations
Weill Cornell Medicine
New York-Presbyterian Hospital
New York, New York, USA

Alexander Ropper, MD
Associate Professor
Baylor College of Medicine
Director of Spinal Neurosurgery
Baylor St. Luke's Medical Center
Houston, Texas, USA

Brain

Achondroplasia

FGFR3 gain-of-function mutation, 20% autosomal dominant and 80% sporadic

Diagnosed by genetic testing, antepartum ultrasound, and familial history

Anatomical features include short pedicles, narrow interpedicular distances, square ilia, narrow sacrosciatic notches, basilar invagination, and spinal stenosis

ETIOLOGY

- Achondroplasia is caused by a gain-of-function mutation in the *FGFR3* gene, which encodes a key regulator of bone growth. This mutation disrupts the proliferation and differentiation of chondrocytes, leading to defects primarily in cartilaginous bone development. As a result, virtually all clinical manifestations of the condition stem from abnormalities in cartilage
- Achondroplasia can be diagnosed prenatally with genetic testing in cases showing ultrasound findings suggestive of the condition and family history, as per the International Achondroplasia Consensus Statement Group. Most cases are diagnosed in infancy. Over 80% of cases are due to sporadic mutations, and advanced paternal age is a known risk factor

FEATURES

- Short stature with rhizomelic disproportion, macrocephaly, thoracolumbar kyphosis, and lumbar hyperlordosis. Skeletal abnormalities include short limbs, short pedicles, narrow interpedicular distances, square ilia, and narrow sacrosciatic notches, along with basilar invagination and spinal stenosis. Hydrocephalus affects 15–50% of individuals

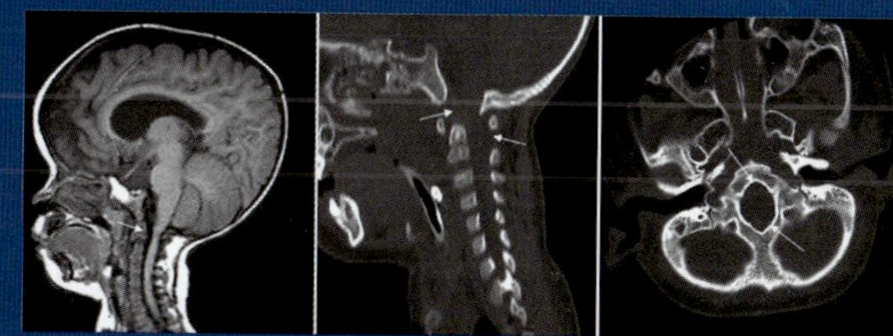

An 8-year-old boy with achondroplasia displaying basilar invagination and cervical spinal stenosis

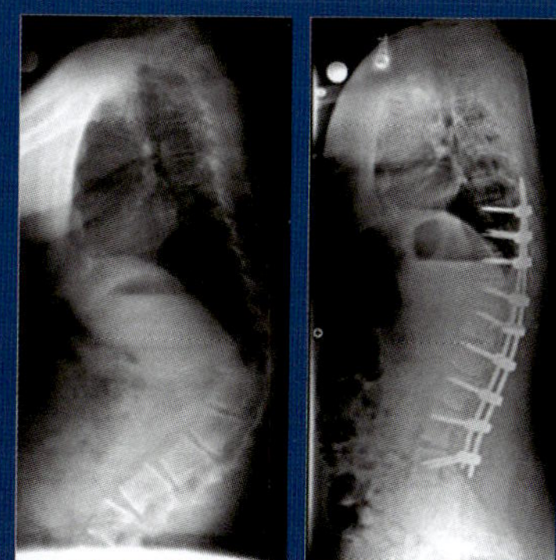

Radiographs of a 17-year-old boy with achondroplasia before and after T8–L4 decompression and fusion indicated for neurogenic claudication

TREATMENT

- Multidisciplinary and lifelong supportive care
- Foramen magnum decompression for cervicomedullary compression in patients with symptomatic myelopathy or syringomyelia, CSF diversion for symptomatic hydrocephalus, and decompression for spinal deformity and stenosis

Further Readings

1. King JA, Vachhrajani S, Drake JM, Rutka JT. Neurosurgical implications of achondroplasia. J Neurosurg Pediatr 2009;4(4):297–306
2. Pauli RM. Achondroplasia: a comprehensive clinical review. Orphanet J Rare Dis 2019 ;14(1):1
3. Greenberg MS. Greenberg's Handbook of Neurosurgery, 10th ed. Thieme Medical Publishing Group; 2023

Nitin Agarwal
David T. Fernandes Cabral
Samuel Adida

Thieme

Acromegaly

Diagnosis is confirmed by measuring elevated IGF-1 and failure to suppress GH after an oral glucose tolerance test

Pharmacologic treatment includes somatostatin analogs, GH receptor antagonists, and dopamine agonists

Neurosurgical intervention consists of gross total surgical resection, and radiotherapy or radiosurgery as adjuvant treatment or as indicated for recurrent disease

PRESENTATION

- Acromegaly is most commonly caused by WHO Grade 1 pituitary somatotroph adenomas. These tumors are classified as microadenomas (<10 mm) or macroadenomas (>10 mm) and are responsible for excessive production of GH
- In adults, excess GH leads to abnormal growth, particularly in the hands, feet, and facial features, while in children, it results in gigantism before the closure of the epiphyseal plates. Genetic factors, such as mutations in MEN1, can increase the likelihood of developing acromegaly
- MRI typically shows well-encapsulated contrast-enhancing masses. Dynamic contrast-enhanced MRI improves the sensitivity for detecting microadenomas

RADIOGRAPHIC FEATURES

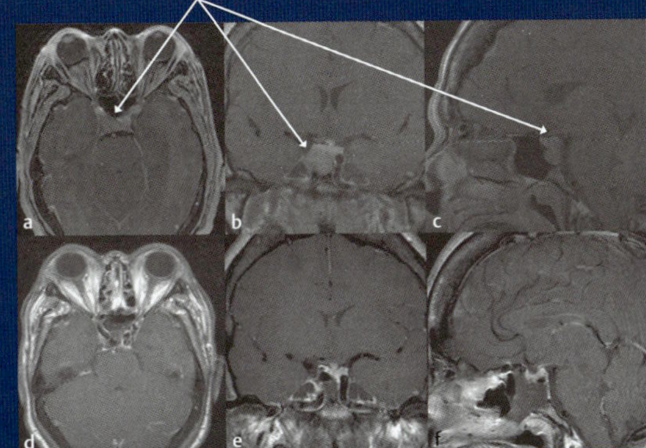

MRI of a 57-year-old patient with acromegaly. Preoperative sequences demonstrate a sellar tumor with extension along the right retrosellar area. Postoperative sequences show resection with use of an endoscopic endonasal approach

TREATMENT

- Pharmacological treatments include somatostatin receptor ligands like octreotide and lanreotide, as well as the GH receptor antagonist pegvisomant. Cabergoline, a dopamine agonist, can be considered in patients with mild acromegaly or those who are resistant to somatostatin analogs
- Transsphenoidal resection is the first-line intervention, offering immediate GH reduction and diagnostic tissue. While surgery often leads to remission, treatment is frequently multimodal. Remission is more likely with lower preoperative GH levels, smaller tumor size, and extra pseudocapsular resection, but macroadenomas and cavernous sinus invasion are linked to lower remission rates
- Radiotherapy is considered for residual or enlarging tumors when surgery and medical treatments fail. Radiosurgery offers similar efficacy to conventional radiotherapy with fewer side effects but has a higher risk of stroke

Further Readings

1. Marquez Y et al. Surgery and radiosurgery for acromegaly: a review of indications, operative techniques, outcomes, and complications. Int J Endocrinol 2012;2012:386–401
2. Zahr R, Fleseriu M. Updates in diagnosis and treatment of acromegaly. Eur Endocrinol 2018;14(2):57–61
3. Greenberg MS. Greenberg's handbook of neurosurgery, 10th ed. Thieme Medical Publishing Group; 2023

Nitin Agarwal
David T. Fernandes Cabral
Samuel Adida

Thieme

Arachnoid Cysts

- Most common intracranial locations are the middle cranial fossa, posterior cranial fossa, and suprasellar region
- The thoracic spine is the most common region for spinal arachnoid cysts

Galassi's classification of arachnoid cysts based on CT and CT cisternography:

- Type I: Small, spindle-shaped cyst in the anterior temporal fossa; no mass effect or midline displacement; communicates with the subarachnoid space
- Type II: Medium-sized, quadrangular cyst extending along the Sylvian fissure; partially communicates with the subarachnoid space
- Type III: Large cyst involving the entire Sylvian fissure, displacing midline structures and compressing frontal and parietal lobes; minimal communication with the subarachnoid space.

PRESENTATION

- Arachnoid cysts are classified as primary developmental cysts or secondary cysts. Primary cysts result from in utero splitting of the arachnoid membranes, leading to CSF accumulation. Secondary cysts develop following trauma, surgery, or infection
- Approximately 95% of patients with arachnoid cysts are asymptomatic, with an average pediatric diagnosis age of 6 years
- The presentation of arachnoid cysts depends on their size and location. Small cysts are typically asymptomatic, while large cysts may cause focal deficits. Arachnoid cysts tend to stop expanding after the age of 4 years
- Symptoms include headache, dizziness, nausea, vomiting, altered mental status, ataxia, seizures, and tinnitus. Rare but notable presentations include intracranial hypertension, visual deterioration, endocrinopathy, and “bobble-head doll syndrome”

RADIOGRAPHIC FEATURES

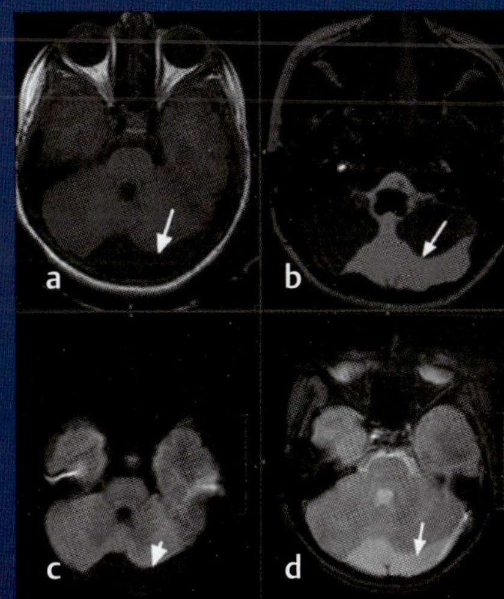

Axial images of the posterior fossa reveal a cerebellar arachnoid cyst exhibiting mass effect. It is hypointense on (a) T1 MRI, hyperintense on (b,d) T2 MRI, and does not exhibit (c) DWI restriction

TREATMENT

- Arachnoid cysts are most commonly located intracranially, with the middle cranial fossa being the predominant site. Other frequent locations include the cerebellopontine angle, suprasellar and quadrigeminal cisterns, cerebral convexities, and cisterna magna. Arachnoid cysts may also occur along the spinal cord
- Arachnoid cysts should be differentiated from epidermoid cysts, which are usually more lobulated and demonstrate diffusion restriction on imaging. In the retrocerebellar space, arachnoid cysts should be differentiated from mega cisterna magna, which does not present with mass effect or contrast enhancement
- Surgical intervention includes microsurgical fenestration via craniotomy, endoscopic fenestration, and cysto-peritoneal shunting

Further Reading

1. Mustansir F, Bashir S, Darbar A. Management of arachnoid cysts: a comprehensive review. Cureus 2018;10(4):e2458
2. Greenberg MS. Greenberg's Handbook of Neurosurgery. 10th ed. Stuttgart, Germany: Thieme Medical Publishing Group; 2023

Nitin Agarwal
David T. Fernandes Cabral
Samuel Adida

Thieme

Arteriovenous Malformations (AVM)

Annual risk of hemorrhage is

1–3%

Genetic risks

- Osler–Weber–Rendu syndrome
- Sturge Weber syndrome
- *KRAS* and *SMAD4/9* mutations

Spetzler-Martin grading scale for arteriovenous malformations

Graded feature	Points
Size	
Small (<3 cm)	1
Medium (3–6 cm)	2
Large (>6 cm)	3
Eloquence of adjacent brain	
Noneloquent	0
Eloquent	1
Draining veins	
Superficial	0
Deep	1

ETIOLOGY

- AVMs are anomalous direct shunts between cerebral arteries and veins that convalesce into a vascular nidus
- Typically, a single feeding artery with a well-defined internal and external elastic lamina. Veins lack an external elastic lamina and have a thin or poorly developed internal elastic lamina

PRESENTATION

- Intracranial AVMs may be identified during the evaluation of strokes, seizures, CN palsies, focal neurological deficits, or incidentally
  - Acute hemorrhage (65%)
  - Seizures (20%)
  - Incidental finding (15%)
  - Focal neurological deficits
    - Ischemic regional "steal" phenomenon
    - Mass effect
  - Pulsatile tinnitus
  - Headache

RADIOGRAPHIC FEATURES

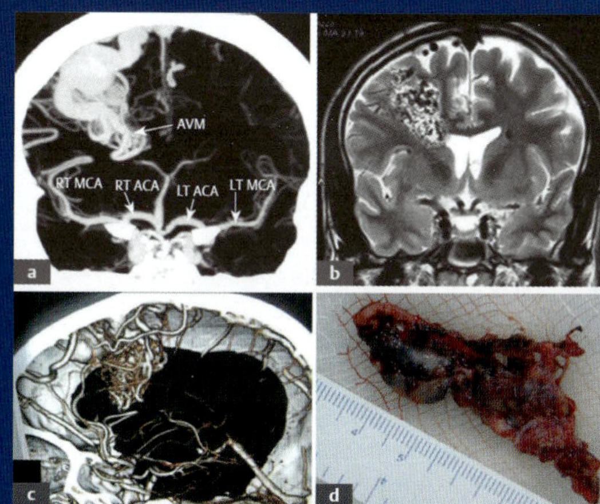

(a) CTA and (b) T2 MRI of a motor cortex AVM. (c) A 3D-reconstructed CTA can better characterize the AVM. (d) Resected specimen

TREATMENT

- The Spetzler–Martin AVM grading scale is used to determine risk of open surgical resection. Resection aims to remove the nidus *en bloc*. High success rates but involves a craniotomy, longer recovery, and higher morbidity. Best for Spetzler–Martin grades I–III, with scores ≤ 6 preferred
- Endovascular embolization controls bleeding, targets simple AVMs, and aids in surgery or SRS. Multi-stage techniques use agents such as onyx and PVA but carry a ~7% risk of complications including hemorrhage and stroke
- SRS is effective for small and medium AVMs in the deep brain structures. Achieves 60–80% obliteration in 3–5 years but risks radiation changes (~36%, symptomatic in ~10%). AVM embolization may negatively affect likelihood of obliteration after SRS
- Ruptured AVMs often require surgery due to high rebleeding risk. The ARUBA and SAIVM trials have investigated outcomes for unruptured AVMs

Further Reading

1. Zyck S, Davidson CL, Sampath R et al. Arteriovenous malformations of the central nervous system. In: StatPearls [Internet]. Treasure Island, FL: StatPearls Publishing; 2024
2. Chen CJ, Ding D, Derdeyn CP et al. Brain arteriovenous malformations: a review of natural history, pathobiology, and interventions. Neurology 2020;95(20):917–927
3. Greenberg MS. Greenberg's Handbook of Neurosurgery. 10th ed. Stuttgart, Germany: Thieme Medical Publishing Group; 2023

Nitin Agarwal
David T. Fernandes Cabral
Samuel Adida

Thieme

Brain Abscesses

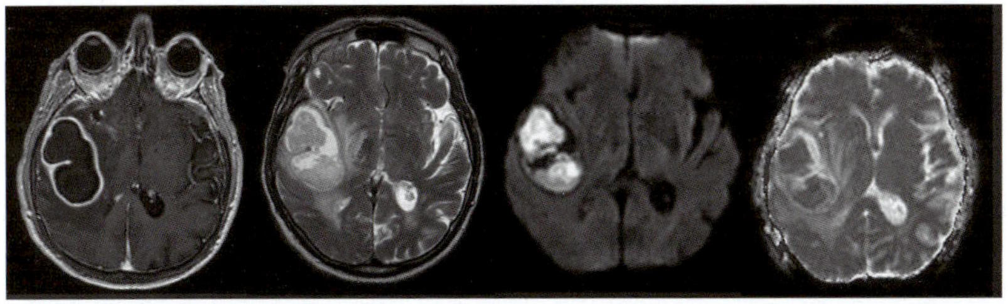

- **Staphylococci spp. and Streptococcus spp. are common in patients with a history of neurosurgery**
- **Staphylococcus spp., Streptococcus spp., Clostridium spp., and Enterobacteriaceae spp. are found in patients with open head trauma**
- **Fungal infections, Toxoplasma gondii, Staphylococcus spp., Streptococcus spp., and Pseudomonas are seen in immunocompromised patients**

PRESENTATION

- Cerebral abscesses are rare, with an estimated 1,500–2,500 cases annually in the United States. Symptoms arise primarily due to increased ICP, including headache, nausea, vomiting, and lethargy. Notably, hemiparesis and seizures occur in 30–50% of cases, with symptom progression typically more rapid than that seen in neoplasms
- Cerebral abscesses commonly result from hematogenous spread of infection, post-surgical complications, or penetrating injuries. They may also occur via contiguous spread (e.g., from frontal sinus or mastoid infections) or, less commonly, through transcoelomic routes (e.g., direct extension through body cavities)
- Seizures and hemiparesis are the most common presenting features. While the classic triad of headache, focal neurological deficit, and fever is often cited, it is observed in only ~20% of patients

RADIOGRAPHIC FEATURES

- On CT with contrast, cerebral abscesses often exhibit a double rim sign, with an outer hypodense and inner hyperdense rim. A uniform, iso-, or hyperdense ring surrounds a hypodense core, with adjacent low-density vasogenic edema
- On MRI, T1 shows a hypointense core with peripheral ring enhancement and surrounding vasogenic edema. On T2/FLAIR, the core appears hyperintense with surrounding edema; the capsule may appear as a thin rim of low signal
- DWI/ADC is key for diagnosis, revealing central diffusion restriction. In immunocompromised patients, this may be absent. SWI highlights the capsule as a smooth low-intensity rim, with the dual rim sign further aiding in diagnosis

TREATMENT

- Blood cultures, WBC count, and β-d-glucan suggest invasive fungal disease. In immunocompromised patients, lab findings alone may support a presumptive diagnosis of *Toxoplasma gondii*. The role of lumbar puncture and CSF analysis may be explored based on the clinical context
- Conservative medical management may suffice for small abscesses without significant mass effect or symptoms
- Management includes biopsy if indicated, and surgical excision or needle aspiration for abscesses near the ventricles. Antimicrobial therapy is essential and may be tailored to the underlying pathogen. Dexamethasone is used to reduce vasogenic edema

Further Reading

1. Bokhari MR, Mesfin FB. Brain abscess. In: StatPearls [Internet]. Treasure Island, FL: StatPearls Publishing; 2024
2. Greenberg MS. Greenberg's Handbook of Neurosurgery. 10th ed. Stuttgart, Germany: Thieme Medical Publishing Group; 2023

Nitin Agarwal
David T. Fernandes Cabral
Samuel Adida

Thieme

Brainstem Cavernoma-Part I

The familial form of CM comprises approximately 6–50% of all cases and are derived from mutations in the CCM1-3 genes

CLINICAL OVERVIEW

Introduction

- Brainstem cavernous malformations (CMs) are low-flow vascular malformations composed of dysplastic capillaries with no normal intervening brain parenchyma. Their deep, eloquent location poses high risk of hemorrhage, leading to significant morbidity even with small-volume bleeds. Surgical intervention is challenging due to their proximity to critical neurovascular structures, necessitating a careful risk–benefit assessment
- The average age of adult presentation is in the fourth or fifth decade of life. Children present in a bimodal pattern with peaks at 0–2 and 13–16 years of age

Pathophysiology

- Thin-walled, leaky vascular channels with hemosiderin deposition, prone to microbleeding and overt hemorrhage
- Most commonly found in the pons (~60%), followed by the midbrain (~20%) and medulla (~15%)
- May be sporadic (single lesion) or familial (multiple lesions), the latter associated with CCM1-3 gene mutations (autosomal dominant inheritance)
- Adjacent developmental venous anomalies (DVAs): Frequently coexist with cavernomas and should be preserved during surgery to avoid venous infarction

Clinical Presentation

- Stepwise neurological decline due to recurrent microhemorrhages
- Focal neurological deficits:
    - Pontine lesions: Hemiparesis, facial weakness, dysarthria, diplopia (CN VI)
    - Midbrain lesions: Oculomotor palsy (CN III), contralateral hemiparesis (Weber's syndrome)
    - Medullary lesions: Dysphagia, vertigo, respiratory dysfunction (lower CN involvement)
- Acute hemorrhage → sudden worsening of symptoms, often requiring urgent intervention
- Seizures are rare, as the brainstem is not epileptogenic

Further Reading

1. Teo C, Sughrue M, eds. Principles and Practice of Keyhole Brain Surgery. 1st ed. Stuttgart: Thieme; 2015

Nitin Agarwal
David T. Fernandes Cabral
Samuel Adida

Thieme

Brainstem Cavernoma-Part II

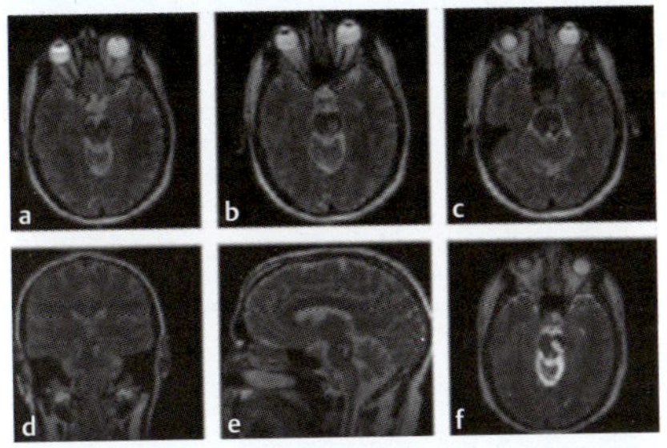

Brainstem cavernomas (BCs) account for 18–35% of CNS cavernomas and can present with hemorrhage or progressive neurological deficit. Approximately 57% of the cavernomas occur in pons followed by midbrain (14%), pontomedullary junction (12%), and medulla (5%).

IMAGING

- MRI is the gold standard: T2weighted imaging:
  - Type I CM contain subacute hemorrhage characterized by a hemosiderin core, which is hyperintense on T1 and T2 sequences
  - Type II CM with loculated areas of hemorrhage are surrounded by gliotic tissue displaying a reticulated mixed signal on appearance
  - Type III lesions, typically seen in familial CM, contain chronic resolved hemorrhage, with T1, T2, and gradient echo sequences displaying an isointense lesion. Familial lesions are also thought to more frequently lack a developmental venous anomaly, which becomes apparent on contrast-enhanced MRI
  - Type IV lesions appear similar to telangiectasias and are only seen on gradient echo MRI as small punctate hypointense signals
- Gradient echo (T2) and SWI (susceptibilityweighted imaging): Most sensitive for detecting hemosiderin deposition from prior hemorrhages
- T1-weighted imaging: Acute hemorrhage may appear hyperintense, while chronic lesions show mixed signal intensities
- FLAIR: May show perilesional edema in active hemorrhage
- CT is typically normal unless a recent hemorrhage is present but lacks specificity
- Catheter angiography is NOT indicated, as cavernomas are angiographically occult

MANAGEMENT

Observation and Serial Imaging
- Indicated for asymptomatic or mildly symptomatic lesions, particularly deep-seated ones
- Follow-up with MRI to assess interval hemorrhage risk

Surgical Resection
- Reserved for symptomatic, recurrent hemorrhages or progressive neurological deterioration
- Operative approach dictated by safest pial or ependymal entry zone to minimize brainstem disruption:
  - Midbrain: Interhemispheric transtentorial or subtemporal approach
  - Pons: Extended retrosigmoid, suboccipital, or lateral supracerebellar-infratentorial approach
  - Medulla: Far-lateral approach
- Intraoperative neuromonitoring is critical due to the high risk of permanent deficit

Stereotactic Radiosurgery (SRS)
- Controversial, generally reserved for deep, inoperable lesions
- Long-term efficacy in hemorrhage reduction remains uncertain

Nitin Agarwal
David T. Fernandes Cabral
Samuel Adida

Thieme

Carotid-Cavernous Fistula-Part I

Direct CCFs are high flow, traumatic, and symptomatic, requiring urgent endovascular treatment, whereas indirect CCFs are low flow and often self-limiting

CLINICAL OVERVIEW

Introduction

- A carotid-cavernous fistula (CCF) is an abnormal connection between the carotid arterial system and the cavernous sinus. This arteriovenous shunting leads to venous congestion, ocular dysfunction, and potential neurological deficits. Early recognition and management are critical to prevent vision loss and intracranial complications

Clinical Presentation

- Classic clinical triad:
    - Pulsatile exophthalmos
    - Conjunctival injection and chemosis ("arterialized" eye)
    - Bruit over the orbit
- Other symptoms:
- Ophthalmoplegia: Cranial nerves III, IV, and VI compression from venous congestion
- Increased intraocular pressure (IOP) → Risk of glaucoma and vision loss
- Cortical venous reflux → Risk of hemorrhage or ischemic stroke (in high-risk fistulas)

Classification

- Type A (direct CCF): High-flow fistula due to direct rupture of the internal carotid artery (ICA) into the cavernous sinus, typically from trauma or aneurysm rupture, requiring urgent intervention
- Type B (indirect CCF): Low-flow fistula arising from meningeal branches of the ICA, often spontaneous or associated with hypertension, with potential for spontaneous resolution or endovascular treatment if symptomatic
- Type C (indirect CCF): Low-flow fistula supplied by meningeal branches of the external carotid artery (ECA), similar to type B in presentation and treatment considerations
- Type D (indirect CCF): Low-flow fistula with dual supply from both ICA and ECA meningeal branches, posing a slightly higher risk of persistent symptoms and requiring closer monitoring or embolization if symptomatic

Further Readings

1. Dahiya A, Dahiya S, Kumar SS, et al. Posttraumatic carotid cavernous fistula: a rare case. Indian J Neurotrauma 2021;18(02):142–145
2. Ellis JA, Goldstein H, Connolly ES Jr, Meyers PM. Carotid-cavernous fistulas. Neurosurg Focus 2012;32(5):E9

Nitin Agarwal
David T. Fernandes Cabral
Samuel Adida

Thieme

Carotid-Cavernous Fistula-Part II

The classic triad—pulsatile proptosis, conjunctival injection, and orbital bruit—should prompt immediate vascular imaging, with digital subtraction angiography (DSA) as the gold standard

CLASSIFICATION

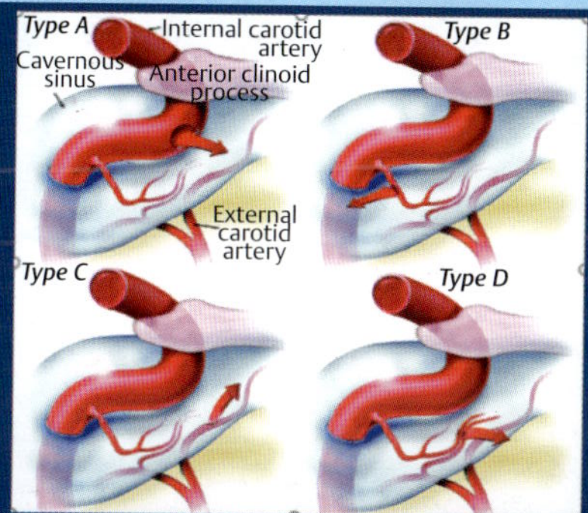

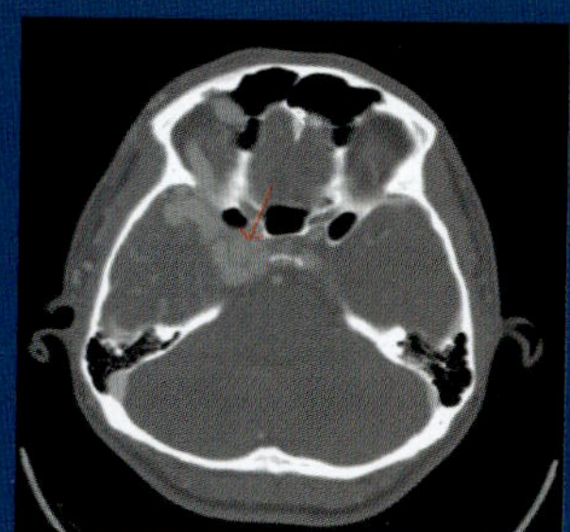

Fistulous communication between
The right intracavernous ICA

Classification of CCF
- CCFs are classified based on their vascular origin and flow dynamics:
- Direct (high-flow) CCF
- Direct communication between the ICA and cavernous sinus
- Typically traumatic or from ICA aneurysm rupture
- High-pressure shunting leads to severe orbital symptoms and cranial nerve dysfunction
- Indirect (low-flow) CCF
- Arise from dural branches of the ECA or ICA
- Often spontaneous, associated with connective tissue disorders or venous hypertension
- More insidious in onset with milder symptoms

Diagnostic Imaging
- CT/MRI with contrast: Cavernous sinus enlargement, proptosis, and enlarged ophthalmic veins
- CT/MR angiography (CTA/MRA) often misses low-flow indirect CCFs, and delayed venous-phase imaging is necessary
- CT/MRA: Noninvasive screening, identifying arterial feeders
- DSA: Gold standard for definitive diagnosis and classification, crucial for treatment planning

Nitin Agarwal
David T. Fernandes Cabral
Samuel Adida

Thieme

Carotid-Cavernous Fistula-Part III

Endovascular embolization is the primary treatment modality, with transvenous access favored for indirect CCFs and transarterial techniques for direct fistulas

MANAGEMENT

Predictors of Spontaneous Resolution

- Indirect (low-flow) CCFs (types B, C, and D)
- Small fistula size
- Mild symptoms: If the patient has minimal proptosis, mild chemosis, or low-grade bruit, the fistula may resolve without intervention
- Venous drainage pattern: If the drainage is primarily anterior (ophthalmic veins) and not into the deep venous system, there is a higher chance of resolution
- Stable or improving symptoms
- No evidence of cortical venous reflux

Predictors Requiring Urgent Intervention

- Direct (high-flow) CCFs (type A): Typically due to traumatic rupture of the ICA into the cavernous sinus, typically require endovascular treatment
- Severe ophthalmologic symptoms: Progressive proptosis, severe chemosis, diplopia, or decreased visual acuity indicate worsening venous congestion
- Cortical venous reflux: Retrograde venous drainage into the cortical veins increases the risk of venous hypertension, intracranial hemorrhage, or seizures
- Intracranial hemorrhage or ischemia
- Elevated IOP leading to glaucoma: Persistent venous congestion can lead to optic neuropathy and vision loss
- Worsening neurologic deficits: If the patient develops cranial nerve palsies (especially CNs III, IV, VI) or progressive neurologic symptoms, intervention is indicated
- High-flow shunting on angiography: Large fistulas with significant arterial supply from the ICA or ECA require intervention to prevent complications

Endovascular Treatment

- Transvenous coil embolization: For indirect CCFs via the inferior petrosal sinus
- Transarterial embolization: For direct CCFs when venous access is limited
- Flow-diverting stents: Emerging therapy for certain direct fistulas
- Surgical ligation: Rarely indicated, reserved for refractory cases or inaccessible fistulas
- Escalate to surgical bypass or ICA trapping if embolization fails and the patient has persistent/worsening symptoms (vision loss, proptosis, cranial nerve deficits), cortical venous reflux with hemorrhage risk, high-flow shunting with arterial steal, recurrent fistula despite multiple embolization attempts, or ICA compromise (stenosis, dissection, pseudoaneurysm)
- *Complications*: Reperfusion hemorrhage, cranial neuropathies post-coil embolization, recurrence, and risk of ICA sacrifice

Postoperative Management

Imaging

- Early (24–48 h postprocedure): CTA or MRA to confirm fistula closure
- Routine (1–3 months posttreatment): Repeat DSA if symptoms persist or there is concern for recurrence
- Long-term (6–12 months): Imaging surveillance, especially for high-risk cases (residual shunting, bypass)

Medical Management

- IOP control: Topical and systemic agents if venous congestion persists
- Anti-inflammatory therapy: Short-term steroids for severe chemosis or orbital inflammation
- Antiplatelet/anticoagulation therapy: If stent-assisted embolization was performed

Nitin Agarwal
David T. Fernandes Cabral
Samuel Adida

Thieme

Cerebrospinal Fluid (CSF) Leaks

May present with orthostatic and positional headaches, nausea and vomiting, neck pain, tinnitus, and cranial nerve deficits like diplopia or hearing loss

β-2 transferrin in rhinorrhea or otorrhea is a highly sensitive and specific marker for CSF

Conservative management includes bed rest and hydration, while lumbar drains and epidural blood patches provide symptom relief; persistent leaks may require nasal packing or primary surgical repair

PRESENTATION

- CSF leaks occur when CSF escapes from the subarachnoid space often due to trauma, surgery, lumbar punctures, or spontaneously
- Symptoms of CSF leaks are primarily due to intracranial hypotension and include orthostatic and positional headaches, dizziness, nausea, vomiting, neck pain, tinnitus, and, in some cases, cranial nerve deficits such as diplopia or hearing loss. Spontaneous CSF leaks may not present with the classic intracranial hypotension syndrome
- Cranial CSF leaks can present with rhinorrhea or otorrhea caused by skull base defects in the cribriform plate, tegmen tympani, or lateral recess of the sphenoid sinus
- Spinal CSF leaks, caused by dural defects such as tears, meningeal diverticula, or CSF-venous fistulas, may result from trauma, surgery, or connective tissue disorders like Marfan's or Ehlers–Danlos syndromes. They present similarly to cranial CSF leaks, and variability in presentation makes diagnosis challenging

RADIOGRAPHIC FEATURES

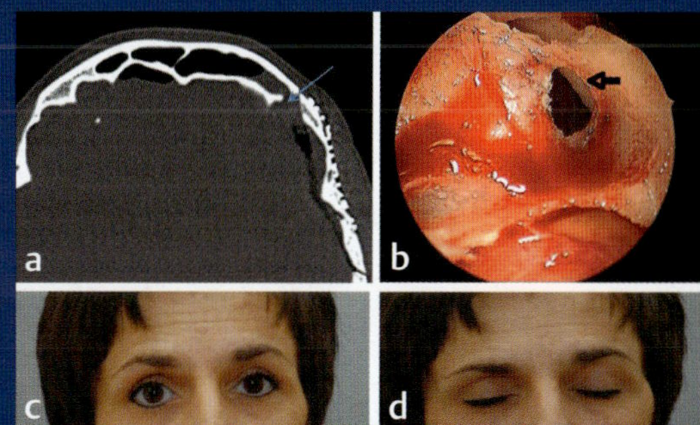

A 42-year-old female who developed a CSF leak following a craniotomy for an aneurysm repair. (a) CT reveals a bony defect in the extreme posterior lateral wall of the frontal sinus. (b) Through a transpalpebral approach, a minifrontal craniotomy was performed and the defect was exposed endoscopically to identify the defect and site of the CSF leak for repair

TREATMENT

- Testing rhinorrhea or otorrhea for β-2 transferrin is a highly specific and sensitive diagnostic tool
- CT or MR myelography may be used to identify the location and underlying cause of a CSF leak. MRI with contrast can reveal pachymeningeal enhancement, subdural fluid collections, venous engorgement, pituitary enlargement, brain sagging, or reduced optic-nerve sheath subarachnoid space volume. However, patients may have normal findings on MRI
- Conservative management includes bed rest and hydration therapy. Lumbar drains temporarily relieve symptoms to give the leak time to mend
- Epidural blood patches can relieve symptoms in most cases. For persistent leaks nasal packing, endoscopic repair, and surgical repair are utilized

Further Reading

1. Severson M, Schaurich CG, Strecker-McGraw MK. Cerebrospinal Fluid Leak. In: StatPearls [Internet]. Treasure Island, FL: StatPearls Publishing; 2024
2. Wang SJ. Spontaneous intracranial hypotension. Continuum (Minneap Minn) 2021;27(3):746–766
3. Greenberg MS. Greenberg's Handbook of Neurosurgery. 10th ed. Stuttgart, Germany: Thieme Medical Publishing Group; 2023

Nitin Agarwal
David T. Fernandes Cabral
Samuel Adida

Thieme

Cerebrovascular Malformations

2–4%
annual hemorrhage risk of arteriovenous malformations

1–8%
annual hemorrhage risk of dural arteriovenous fistulas

1%
annual hemorrhage risk of cavernous malformations

PRESENTATION

- Arteriovenous malformations (AVMs):
  - AVMs are direct connections between arteries and veins without an intervening capillary bed, leading to high-flow, low-resistance shunts
  - They are associated with hereditary hemorrhagic telangiectasia (Osler–Weber–Rendu syndrome), an autosomal dominant disorder
  - AVMs may present with headaches, seizures, or neurological deficits; however, they often remain asymptomatic until rupture
- Dural arteriovenous fistulas (dAVFs):
  - dAVFs involve abnormal connections between dural arteries and dural venous sinuses or cortical veins
  - While many dAVFs are sporadic or iatrogenic after cranial or spine surgery, they are associated with Foix–Alajouanine syndrome
  - Symptoms may include headaches, pulsatile tinnitus, visual disturbances, or neurological deficits due to venous hypertension
- Cavernous malformations (CMs):
  - CMs are clusters of abnormal and hyalinized capillaries without intervening brain tissue
  - CMs may occur sporadically or in association with syndromes such as Sturge–Weber syndrome
  - They may present with seizures, focal neurological deficits, or hemorrhage; the risk of bleeding is generally lower than that of AVMs and dAVFs

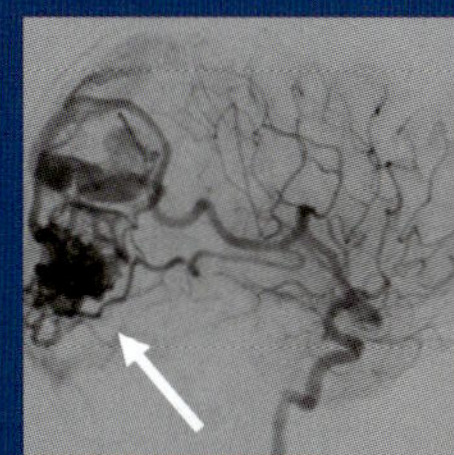
DSA showing a grade V AVM with feeders from the left MCA

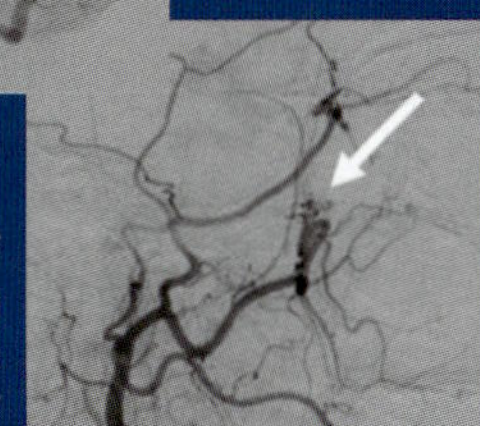
DSA of a dAVF of the sphenopalatine artery

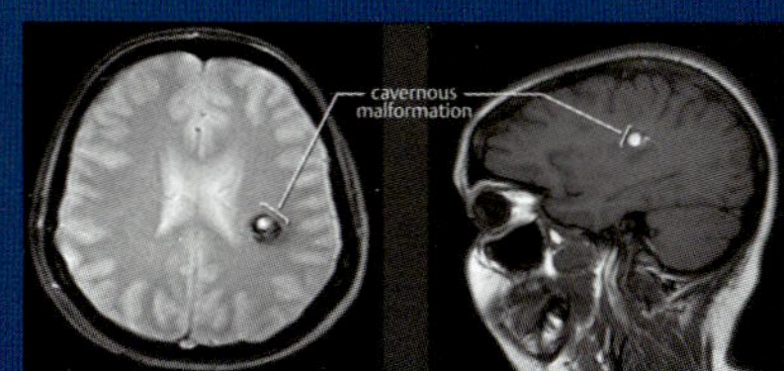

CMs are angiogram negative; depicted is an MRI of a L hemisphere CM

TREATMENT

- Conservative treatment for AVMs includes BP control to reduce rupture risk and antiepileptics to manage seizures or encephalopathy. Intervention includes microsurgical resection, endovascular embolization, and SRS, with the choice of treatment guided by Spetzler–Martin grading
- Low-grade dAVFs, such as Cognard types I–IIa or Borden type I, generally require no intervention unless symptomatic, as they carry a low risk of hemorrhage. High-grade dAVFs, such as Cognard types IIb–V or Borden types II–III, pose a significant risk of complications and are treated with microsurgical resection, endovascular embolization, or SRS
- For CMs, asymptomatic lesions are managed conservatively, while symptomatic cases, particularly those with recurrent hemorrhage, are treated with microsurgical resection. In cases associated with Sturge–Weber syndrome, management also addresses seizures, genetic counseling, and systemic manifestations

Further Readings

1. Mouchtouris N, Chalouhi N, Chitale A, et al. Management of cerebral cavernous malformations: from diagnosis to treatment. ScientificWorldJournal 2015;2015:808314
2. Greenberg MS. Greenberg's Handbook of Neurosurgery. 10th ed. New York, NY: Thieme Medical Publishing Group; 2023

Nitin Agarwal
David T. Fernandes Cabral
Samuel Adida

Thieme

Chiari Malformations

PRESENTATION

- Chiari I malformation:
  - Characterized by the descent of the cerebellar tonsils >5 mm below the foramen magnum
  - Associated with a small posterior cranial fossa, leading to obstructive hydrocephalus presenting with Valsalva-induced suboccipital headaches. Syrinx, or a cystic cavity in the spinal cord, may be present in 27–66% of cases, potentially causing hand weakness, decreased pain and temperature sensation, and incontinence
  - Associated with connective tissue disorders such as Ehlers–Danlos syndrome, and may coexist with idiopathic intracranial hypertension or tethered cord syndrome

- Chiari II malformation:
  - Involves descent of the cerebellar vermis and fourth ventricle below the foramen magnum. Strongly associated with open neural tube defects, typically myelomeningocele
  - Symptoms are often present at birth or in infancy and include difficulty swallowing, stridor, apnea, and weakness. Hydrocephalus and other CN deficits are common
  - May also be linked to other congenital skeletal abnormalities

- Chiari III–V malformations:
  - Rare and severe forms of Chiari malformation, with distinct anatomical abnormalities:
    - Chiari III: Occipital encephalocele with displacement of cerebellar structures into the defect
    - Chiari IV: Cerebellar hypoplasia without herniation
    - Chiari V: Cerebellar hypoplasia with ectopia of the occipital lobe into the posterior fossa
  - Typically diagnosed in neonates or fetuses, and are often fatal or result in severe disability, with symptoms reflecting profound neurological dysfunction

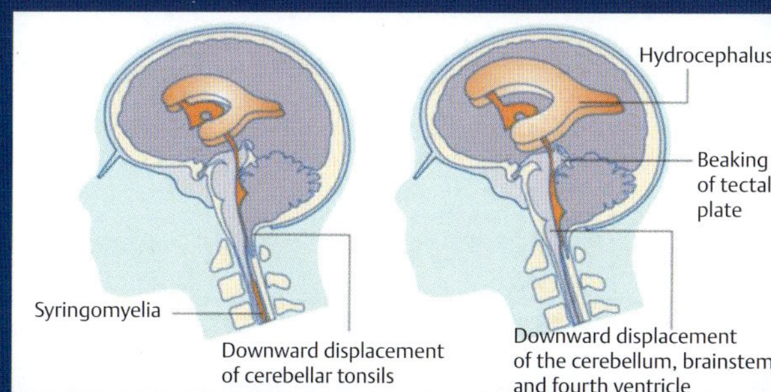

- **Chiari I: Cerebellar tonsils >5 mm below the foramen magnum, causes Valsalva-induced headaches and hydrocephalus; associated with syrinx, connective tissue disorders, and tethered cord syndrome**
- **Chiari II: Descent of the cerebellar vermis and fourth ventricle below the foramen magnum; primarily presents in children and is associated with myelomeningocele**

TREATMENT

- Chiari I malformation:
  - Asymptomatic cases with no syrinx require observation only
  - Symptomatic cases may benefit from posterior fossa decompression, which restores CSF flow and alleviates pressure on the cervicomedullary junction
  - In cases with syringomyelia, duraplasty and cerebellar tonsil reduction may be performed

- Chiari II malformation:
  - Management often requires a multidisciplinary approach
  - Early surgical correction of myelomeningocele is standard
  - Hydrocephalus is managed with ventricular shunting, while posterior fossa decompression may alleviate severe brainstem compression

Further Readings

1. Friedlander RM. Congenital and acquired Chiari syndrome. N Engl J Med 2024;390(23):2191–2198
2. Piper RJ, Pike M, Harrington R, Magdum SA. Chiari malformations: principles of diagnosis and management. BMJ 2019;365:l1159
3. Greenberg MS. Greenberg's Handbook of Neurosurgery. 10th ed. New York, NY: Thieme Medical Publishing Group; 2023

Nitin Agarwal
David T. Fernandes Cabral
Samuel Adida

Thieme

Chondrosarcomas

- **Chondrosarcoma of the skull base and spine are rare, as they commonly arise in the appendicular skeleton such as the pelvis**
- **En bloc resection with wide margins and postoperative high-dose RT is the mainstay treatment**
- **Recurrence rates range from 5 to 39% after surgery alone and 2 to 43% with postoperative radiotherapy**

ETIOLOGY

- Chondrosarcoma is a malignant tumor from mesenchymal cells or cartilaginous matrix remnants, and the second most common primary bone cancer after osteosarcoma. It is rare in the skull base and spine, commonly arising in the appendicular skeleton, such as the pelvis
- Skull base chondrosarcomas typically arise in the clivus, petrous, and sphenoid bones, presenting with headaches, CN deficits, visual disturbances, and hearing loss. Due to slow growth, symptoms are often subtle, leading to delayed diagnosis. Advanced cases may cause severe CN deficits
- Spinal chondrosarcoma, most often occurring in the thoracic spine, presents with localized pain, radicular pain, sensory and motor deficits, bladder and bowel dysfunction, and gait abnormalities

RADIOGRAPHIC FEATURES

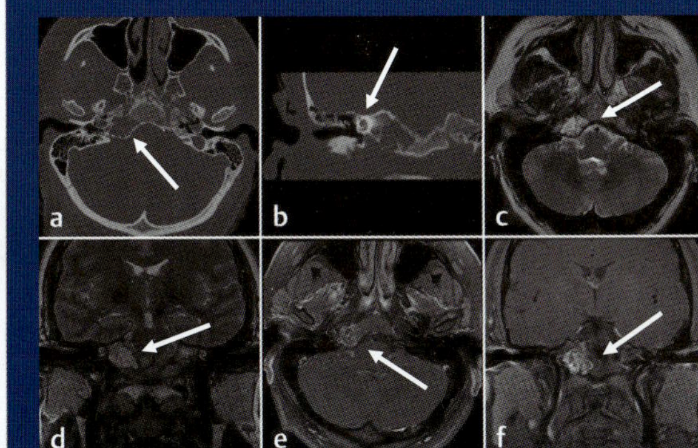

(a, b) Preoperative CT shows a R petroclival chondrosarcoma. MRI shows (c, d) hyperintensity on T2 and (e, f) enhancement after contrast on T1

TREATMENT

- Chondrosarcomas are categorized into conventional, myxoid, mesenchymal, and dedifferentiated subtypes. Conventional chondrosarcoma is slow growing and low grade, while mesenchymal and dedifferentiated subtypes are aggressive with poorer outcomes
- Mainstay treatment for chondrosarcoma is en bloc resection with wide margins, although complete resection may be challenging due to nerve and vascular involvement
- Chondrosarcomas are radioresistant, requiring high-dose RT postresection to reduce recurrence
- Chemotherapy is generally ineffective, except for aggressive subtypes that may respond to combined chemotherapy and RT
- Due to high recurrence and metastasis risk, long-term imaging surveillance is essential

Further Readings

1. Palmisciano PA, Haider AS, Sabahi M et al. Primary skull base chondrosarcomas: a systematic review. Cancers (Basel) 2021;13(23):5960
2. Arshi A, Sharim J, Park DY, et al. Chondrosarcoma of the osseous spine: an analysis of epidemiology, patient outcomes, and prognostic factors using the seer registry from 1973 to 2012. Spine (Phila Pa 1976) 2017;42(9):644–652
3. Ravindran PK, Keizer ME, Kunst HDPM et al. Skull-base chondrosarcoma: a systematic review of the role of postoperative radiotherapy. Cancers (Basel) 2024;16(5):856

Nitin Agarwal
David T. Fernandes Cabral
Samuel Adida

Thieme

Choroid Plexus Tumors

<1%
of all intracranial tumors

Present with symptoms of increased ICP secondary to obstructive hydrocephalus including headache, nausea, and vomiting, and may present along with subarachnoid hemorrhage, seizures, and focal neurological deficits

Gross tumor resection is typically curative, and recurrence is rare

ETIOLOGY

- The choroid plexus is a lobulated structure located within the ventricles and plays a critical role in producing CSF and maintaining the blood-CSF barrier
- Originating from neuroectodermal tissue, the choroid plexus can give rise to a spectrum of tumors including choroid plexus papillomas (WHO grade 1), atypical choroid plexus papillomas (WHO grade 2), and choroid plexus carcinomas (WHO grade 3)
- Neonatal choroid plexus papillomas are thought to be congenital, with some studies suggesting an association with viral infections
- Patients present with symptoms of obstructive hydrocephalus, such as headache, nausea, vomiting, and lethargy. Additional presentations may include meningismus caused by subarachnoid hemorrhage, seizures, and focal neurological deficits

RADIOGRAPHIC FEATURES

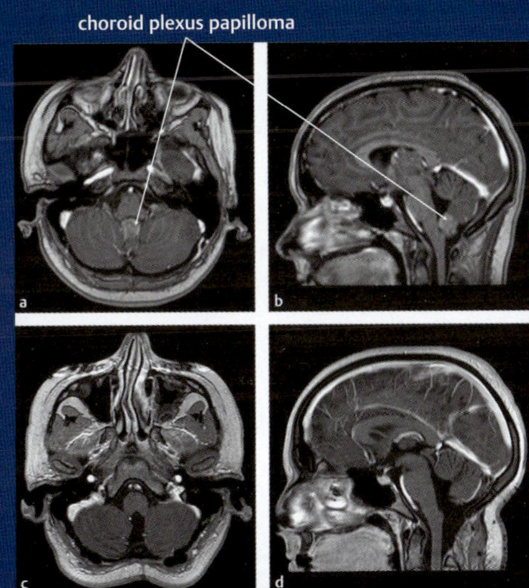

(a,b) Preoperative and (c,d) postoperative MRI of a choroid plexus papilloma arising in the fourth ventricle that underwent tumor resection

TREATMENT

- Imaging studies can assist in diagnosis and surgical planning; CT reveals isodense or hyperdense intraventricular lesions accompanied by ventriculomegaly, and MRI shows a well-defined, lobulated mass
- Gross tumor resection is the treatment of choice in symptomatic patients and is typically curative; recurrence is rare
- Choroid plexus tumors are globular, friable pink masses with irregular projections and are highly vascularized. Pediatric perioperative mortality following resection is 12% due to catastrophic hemorrhage, and preoperative tumor embolization can minimize this risk
- Adjuvant chemotherapy has been shown to prevent recurrence and prolong survival in select patients. Radiosurgery is a possible treatment option

References
1. Joseph JJ, Weisbrod LJ, Das JM. Choroid Plexus Papilloma. In: StatPearls [Internet]. Treasure Island, FL: StatPearls Publishing; 2024
2. Greenberg MS. Greenberg's Handbook of Neurosurgery. 10th ed. Stuttgart, Germany: Thieme Medical Publishing Group; 2023

Nitin Agarwal
David T. Fernandes Cabral
Samuel Adida

Thieme

Clival Chordomas

- **En bloc resection with wide margins is the traditional standard of care, though complete resection is difficult to achieve and often complicated**
- **It is a radioresistant tumor and typically treated with high-dose RT, proton beam, carbon ion, or SRS after resection**
- **5-, 10-, and 15-year recurrence rates of ~30, ~45, and ~60%, respectively**

PRESENTATION

- Chordomas are slow-growing, low-grade, and locally invasive tumors arising from remnants of the notochord. Most commonly found in the sacrum (50%), followed by the skull base (35%) and mobile spine (15%)
- Primarily affect individuals aged 40–60 years, with a male-to-female ratio of 2:1. Symptoms vary by location; clival chordomas may cause headaches, CN dysfunction, or CSF leaks
- Differential diagnosis:
    - Chordomas make up most clival tumors, but clival masses in patients with cancer are more likely metastases
    - Ecchordosis physaliphora is histopathologically indistinguishable from chordoma, but does not demonstrate contrast enhancement
    - Chondrosarcomas are often more laterally situated compared to chordomas, which are more midline, and definitive diagnosis requires biopsy

RADIOGRAPHIC FEATURES

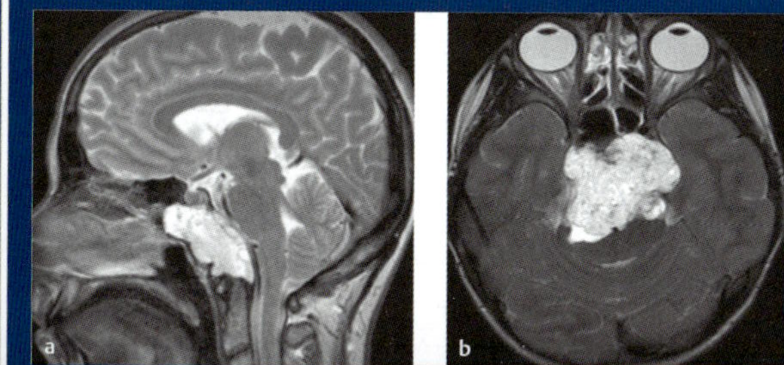

MRI showing a clival chordoma

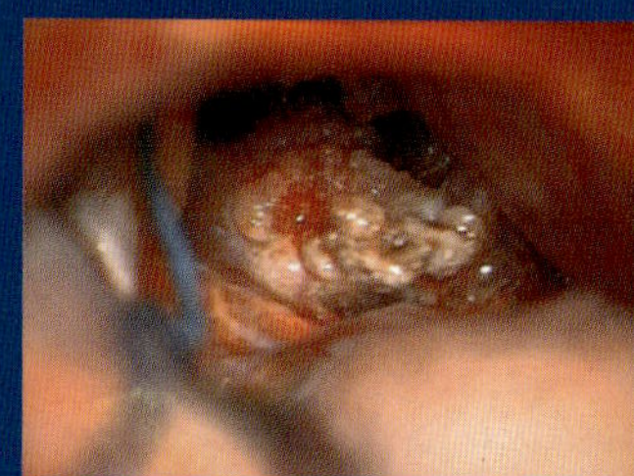

Intraoperative image showing a clival chordoma prior to resection

TREATMENT

- Primary treatment:
    - Surgical resection, ideally en bloc with wide margins, is the mainstay treatment
    - Intralesional resection is effective when coupled with adjuvant RT
- RT:
    - High-dose RT is required due to radioresistance and high recurrence rates
    - Modalities such as proton beam therapy, carbon ion therapy, and SRS may be preferred for their precision and tissue-sparing benefits. They may also serve as primary or definitive treatments when surgery is contraindicated
- Chemotherapy:
    - Generally not effective
- Prognosis and surveillance:
    - Imaging surveillance is critical to monitor for progression or metastasis
    - 5-year survival rate is ~50%, with outcomes depending on tumor size, location, and extent of surgical and adjuvant treatment

Further Readings

1. Baier MP, Cheong DA, Shi HH, et al. Decision-making in clival mass lesions: risk factors for malignant disease and an illustrative case example. J Neurol Surg Rep 2023;84(4):e156–e162
2. Stacchiotti S, Gronchi A, Fossati P, et al. Best practices for the management of local-regional recurrent chordoma: a position paper by the Chordoma Global Consensus Group. Ann Oncol 2017;28(6):1230–1242
3. Tenny S, Varacallo MA. Chordoma. Treasure Island, FL: StatPearls Publishing; 2025

Nitin Agarwal
David T. Fernandes Cabral
Samuel Adida

Thieme

Colloid Cysts

<1%
of all intracranial tumors

The characteristic obstructive hydrocephalus affecting only the lateral ventricles, while sparing the third and fourth ventricles, is pathognomonic

- **Complete resection is curative, with approaches including transcallosal, transcortical, transventricular, and endoscopic approaches**
- **Shunting involves bilateral ventricular shunts**

ETIOLOGY

- Colloid cysts are rare, benign tumors typically found in the anterior third ventricle, occurring in ~3.2 per 1 million persons annually
- May present with hydrocephalus and increased ICP, leading to symptoms like headache, papilledema, nausea, vomiting, visual deficits, dizziness, ataxia, cognitive decline, and seizures
- Differential diagnoses include basilar artery aneurysms, hamartomas, malignancy, choroid plexus papilloma, central neurocytoma, intraventricular meningioma, and ependymomas
- Imaging shows cysts in the third ventricle, blocking both foramina of Monro. On T1 MRI, a majority of colloid cysts are hyperintense. On T2, most are isointense with some showing peripheral rim enhancement. Colloid cysts do not exhibit diffusion restriction

RADIOGRAPHIC FEATURES

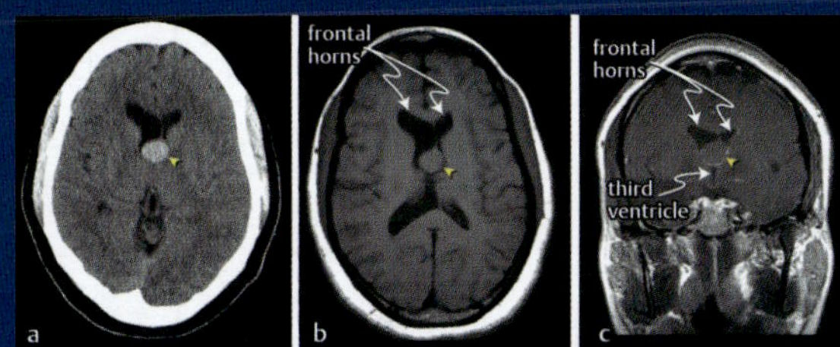

(a) Noncontrast CT, (b) T1 FLAIR MRI, and (c) T1 contrast-enhanced MRI show the relation of the normal-sized third ventricle to the enlarged frontal horns of the lateral ventricles. In this patient, only the right lateral ventricle is enlarged

OTHER CONSIDERATIONS

- Histopathologically, they are unilocular and filled with viscous material. The cell wall is unicellular, typically composed of columnar epithelium, which may or may not be ciliated, with a hypocellular and fibrous stroma
- Most cysts are positive for low- and high-molecular-weight cytokeratins, and immunohistochemistry is negative for prealbumin, neuron-specific enolase, S100 protein, and GFAP

TREATMENT

- Optimal treatment for colloid cysts remains controversial. Surgical options, when indicated, include transcallosal, transcortical, transventricular, and endoscopic approaches
- While complete surgical resection is curative, recurrence is possible. Shunting, which involves bilateral ventricular shunts, may alleviate symptoms but carries the risks of shunt dependency and potential tumor progression

Further Readings

1. Greenberg MS. Greenberg's Handbook of Neurosurgery. 10th ed. New York, NY: Thieme Medical Publishing Group; 2023

Nitin Agarwal
David T. Fernandes Cabral
Samuel Adida

Thieme

Craniopharyngiomas

Adam and papillary mutations

Presenting symptoms panhypopit

Management includes open or EEA resection ± conventional RT or SRS

ETIOLOGY

- Craniopharyngiomas are benign tumors (~25% sellar, ~75% suprasellar) that often involve the hypothalamus, optic chiasm, and CNs. While more common in children, they can occur at any age. They are classified into adamantinomatous and papillary subtypes. Adamantinomatous craniopharyngiomas, which are more common and affect all age groups, tend to be cystic, with solid, cystic, and calcified components. Papillary craniopharyngiomas are mostly seen in adults and are often noncalcified and solid
- Symptoms are related to tumor location and include headache, visual deficits (such as bitemporal hemianopsia), and panhypopituitarism. Other signs can include endocrine deficiency, growth failure, and hypothalamic deficiency like obesity or temperature regulation issues. MRI typically shows a heterogeneous tumor with solid, cystic, and calcified components
- Differential diagnoses include Rathke's cleft cyst, pituitary macroadenoma, pituitary apoplexy, and germ cell tumors

RADIOGRAPHIC FEATURES

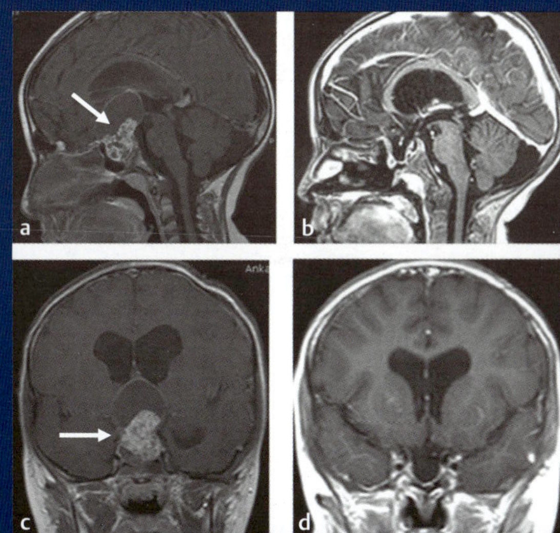

(a, c) Preoperative and (b, d) postoperative MRI of a 5-year-old boy with a craniopharyngioma

TREATMENT

- Evaluation for hormonal deficiencies is essential, involving testing for AM cortisol, ACTH, TSH, free T4, FSH, estradiol or testosterone, GH, IGF-1, prolactin, serum Na, and urine-specific gravity and osmolality. Hormonal deficiency should be treated with HRT
- Management includes open or EEA resection and conventional RT or SRS. Mortality ranges from 5 to 10%, mostly from hypothalamic injury; 5-year survival ranges from 55 to 85%

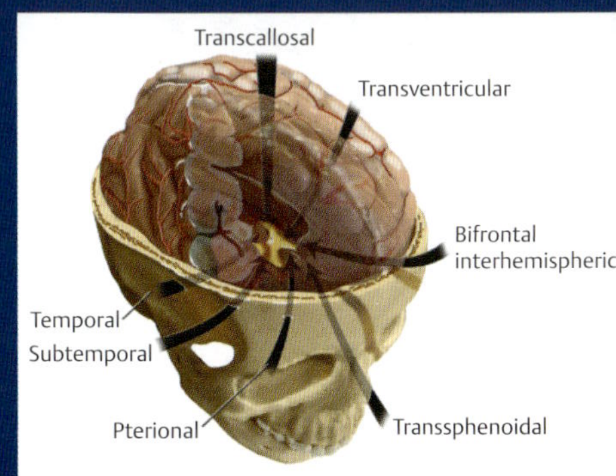

Further Readings

1. Ortiz Torres M, Shafiq I, Mesfin FB. Craniopharyngioma. Treasure Island, FL: StatPearls Publishing; 2024
2. Greenberg MS. Greenberg's Handbook of Neurosurgery. 10th ed. New York, NY: Thieme Medical Publishing Group; 2023

Nitin Agarwal
David T. Fernandes Cabral
Samuel Adida

Thieme

Cushing's Disease

Cushing's disease accounts for

80%

of all endogenous Cushing's syndromes

- **Surgical resection is the mainstay treatment for ACTH-secreting pituitary adenomas, achieving endocrine remission in 69–90% of cases. Common complications include hypopituitarism, diabetes insipidus, and CSF leak, as well as rare complications such as vascular or neural injury. Recurrence rates range from 9 to 30%**
- **SRS is often used for incompletely resected adenomas, achieving endocrine remission in 35–72% of cases. The most common complication of SRS is a new anterior pituitary deficiency, and recurrence ranges from 18 to 24%**

ETIOLOGY

- Cushing's syndrome is a constellation of findings caused by hypercortisolism. There are two etiologies of Cushing's syndrome, endogenous and exogenous hypercortisolism. Cushing's disease is ACTH-dependent cortisol excess due to a pituitary adenoma

PRESENTATION

- Patients may present with weight gain, fatigue weakness, bone pain, loss of height, depression or emotional reactivity, loss of libido, irregular menstrual cycles, infertility, hirsutism, or visual deficit including bitemporal hemianopia
- Pituitary microadenoma in a 27-year-old female

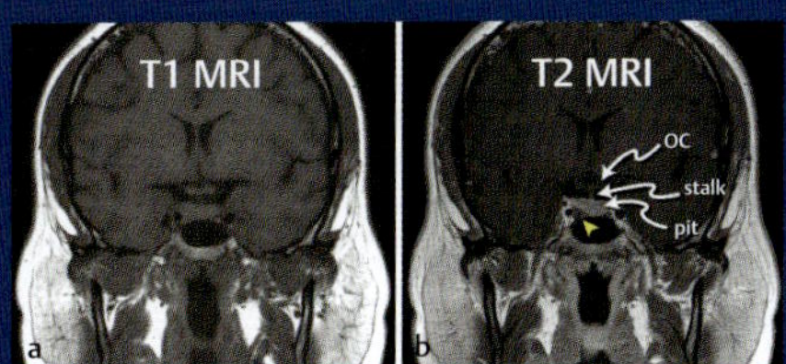

DIAGNOSIS

- Initial evaluation for hypercortisolism:
  - Late-night salivary cortisol or 24-h urine free cortisol assesses dysregulated circadian rhythm and excessive cortisol production
  - Low-dose dexamethasone suppression test confirms autonomous cortisol production, distinguishing Cushing's syndrome from stress-related hypercortisolism
- Determining etiology with serum ACTH:
  - ACTH dependent: Elevated ACTH indicates Cushing's disease (pituitary adenoma) or ectopic ACTH secretion
  - ACTH independent: Low ACTH suggests adrenal adenomas or other adrenal causes
- Further differentiation:
  - High-dose dexamethasone suppression test distinguishes Cushing's disease (suppression occurs) from ectopic ACTH production (nonsuppressible)

TREATMENT

- Surgical treatment typically involves an endoscopic endonasal transsphenoidal approach, with ipsilateral medial wall resection via a transcavernous approach if the tumor invades the cavernous sinus
- For incomplete resection or recurrence, re-resection or SRS should be considered
- Postoperative management includes monitoring for adrenal insufficiency and glucocorticoid replacement until adrenal function recovers
- Pharmacological treatment:
  - Indicated for nonsurgical candidates and those with residual disease
    - Pasireotide: Somatostatin analog
    - Cabergoline: Dopamine agonist
    - Mifepristone: Glucocorticoid receptor antagonist
    - Ketoconazole and metyrapone: Inhibit adrenal steroidogenesis; used as adjunctive therapies

Further Readings

1. Chaudhry HS, Singh G. Cushing Syndrome. Treasure Island, FL: StatPearls Publishing; 2024
2. Bunevicius A, Laws ER , Vance ML, Iuliano S, Sheehan J. Surgical and radiosurgical treatment strategies for Cushing's disease. J Neurooncol 2019;145(3):403–413
3. Tritos N, Biller BMK, Swearingen B. Management of Cushing disease. Nat Rev Endocrinol 2011;7, 279–289
4. Greenberg MS. Greenberg's Handbook of Neurosurgery. 10th ed. New York, NY: Thieme Medical Publishing Group; 2023

Nitin Agarwal
David T. Fernandes Cabral
Samuel Adida

Thieme

Decompressive Hemicraniectomy-Part I

DHC is indicated in patients with refractory intracranial hypertension (>20–25 mm Hg) from TBI or stroke despite maximal medical management, particularly when there is impending brain herniation

OVERVIEW

- Decompressive hemicraniectomy (DHC) is a neurosurgical procedure that involves the removal of a portion of the skull to allow for the expansion of the brain and reduce elevated intracranial pressure (ICP) due to conditions such as traumatic brain injury (TBI), ischemic stroke, or intracranial hemorrhage
- The procedure is typically performed in patients who demonstrate refractory ICP despite maximal medical management

DHC is primarily indicated in situations where there is a risk of brain herniation due to increased ICP, particularly when conservative measures fail to control the pressure. Key indications include the following:

- Malignant cerebral edema following severe TBI or ischemic stroke
- Intracranial hemorrhage: Particularly large subdural hematomas or intraparenchymal hemorrhages with significant mass effect and swelling
- Postcardiac arrest: After a global ischemic insult resulting in cerebral edema
- Pediatric indications: Often performed in children with TBI or stroke, where the brain has a higher capacity for postsurgical recovery

Surgical Indication

- Glasgow Coma Scale (GCS) ≤ 8: Severe TBI with neurological deterioration despite medical management
- ICP > 20–25 mm Hg refractory to medical therapy: Persistent elevated ICP despite hyperosmolar therapy (mannitol, hypertonic saline), sedation, and CSF drainage
- Signs of herniation: Uncal herniation (blown pupil, contralateral hemiparesis), central herniation (bilateral fixed pupils, decerebrate posturing), or tonsillar herniation (irregular respirations, hemodynamic instability)
- Large hemispheric infarct or contusion with midline shift > 5 mm: Significant mass effect with impending herniation
- Refractory or worsening neurological status: Progressive decline despite aggressive ICU management

Nitin Agarwal
David T. Fernandes Cabral
Samuel Adida

Thieme

Decompressive Hemicraniectomy-Part II

Early intervention (within 24 h of injury) improves survival rates, though functional outcomes depend on the severity of brain injury and patient factors

SURGICAL TECHNIQUE

Preoperative Considerations
- Assess the severity of brain swelling and ICP levels (intraventricular catheters or fiberoptic ICP monitors)
- Radiographic assessment:
    - Rotterdam CT score of TBI
    - Marshall classification of TBI
- Ideally, DHC is performed immediately, once patient fails maximal medical management

Surgical Procedure
- Skin incision: A large, reverse question mark scalp incision is made over the area of the brain that is most affected (usually the frontotemporal area, although occipital or parietal regions may also be considered)
- Bone flap removal: The cranium is exposed, and a large bone flap (~12–15 cm) is removed, often in a crescent shape, to provide adequate space for brain expansion
- Dura mater incision: The dura is opened or left intact, depending on the degree of swelling and the need for further decompression. In some cases, a duraplasty may be required

Postoperative care: The bone flap is typically stored in a sterile container (or in the patient's abdomen for later reimplantation) for later cranioplasty once the swelling has resolved

Postoperative Management
- ICP monitoring
- Monitor flap consistency (soft)
- Neuroprotective strategies: These may include sedation, analgesia, and hyperosmolar therapy (e.g., mannitol or hypertonic saline) to further reduce ICP
- Seizure prophylaxis
- Ventilator management: Rehabilitation—Begin rehabilitation as soon as the patient is stable, including early mobilization, physical therapy, and neuropsychological support

Nitin Agarwal
David T. Fernandes Cabral
Samuel Adida

Thieme

Decompressive Hemicraniectomy-Part III

A large bone flap (typically frontotemporoparietal, 15 cm X 12 cm) is required to ensure adequate decompression, with duraplasty often performed to further reduce ICP

POSTOPERATIVE

Complications: While DHC is life-saving in many instances, it carries potential complications. Postoperative ICP monitoring is essential

- Hydrocephalus: Major concern, monitored with ICP monitors, serial imaging, and clinical examination
- Re-expansion syndrome: Brain tissue swells too quickly after decompression, often in the first 72 h after surgery
- Infection: Including wound infections or meningitis, monitored with serial labs and clinical examination
- Seizures: Can occur, particularly in patients with TBI or intracranial hemorrhage, postoperative AED prophylaxis
- Cerebral herniation: Although the goal is to relieve ICP, improper surgical technique or delayed decompression can exacerbate herniation
- Cranial deformities: After bone flap removal, cranial deformities can occur, especially if the flap is not reimplanted in a timely manner

Outcomes: The effectiveness of DHC in improving outcomes is well documented, especially in cases of severe TBI and stroke. Key outcomes depend on the following:

- Timing: Early intervention (within 24–48 h) improves the likelihood of functional recovery
- Patient age and comorbidities
- Initial GCS score
- Postoperative rehabilitation

Long-Term Management

- Reimplantation of the bone flap: Usually performed 3–6 months postsurgery once the brain has had time to heal and swelling has resolved. The decision to reimplant depends on the patient's neurological recovery and any imaging findings (such as resolution of edema)
- Cranioplasty: If reimplantation is not possible due to bone flap loss or infection, custom titanium or other prosthetic cranioplasties can be used to restore the cranial vault

Nitin Agarwal
David T. Fernandes Cabral
Samuel Adida

Thieme

Diffuse Intrinsic Pontine Gliomas

10–15%

of pediatric brain tumors

Classic symptom triad
- **Cranial neuropathy**
- **Motor weakness**
- **Cerebellar signs**

- **Median age at diagnosis is six years**
- **Median survival of nine months**
- **Two-year survival is 10%**
- **Five-year survival is less than 1%**

PRESENTATION

- Diffuse intrinsic pontine glioma (DIPG) is a highly aggressive pediatric brain tumor that arises in the ventral pons. It is the second most common malignant pediatric brain tumor and the leading cause of childhood brain tumor-related deaths
- DIPG progresses rapidly, with most children experiencing symptoms within a month before diagnosis. Roughly 50% of patients will display a classic triad of:
    - Diplopia or facial weakness and asymmetry due to CN VI or CN VII neuropathies
    - Extremity weakness, hyperreflexia, and Babinski sign due to involvement of the corticospinal tract
    - Ataxia, dysmetria, or dysarthria due to cerebellar involvement
- Dorsal tumor extension can cause obstructive hydrocephalus in 10% of cases, leading to increased ICP, headache, nausea, fatigue, and obtundation

RADIOGRAPHIC FEATURES

- Diagnosis relies on clinical history and characteristic MRI findings:
    - Diffuse infiltration of the pons
    - Poor tumor demarcation
    - Basilar artery involvement
    - Lack of gadolinium enhancement

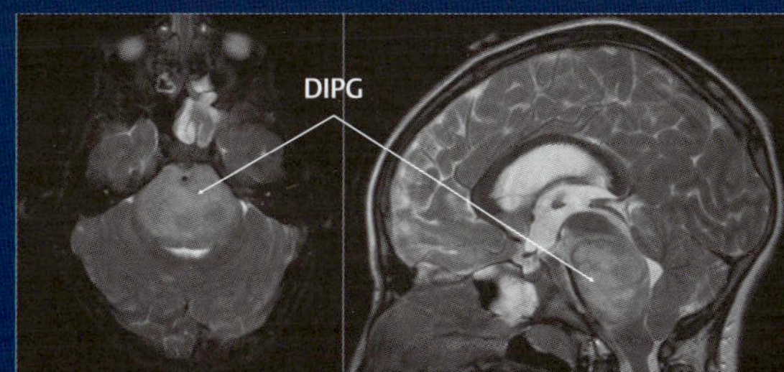

Description of T2 MRI of a DIPG

TREATMENT

- Due to its diffuse growth and infiltration of critical brainstem structures, DIPG cannot be resected
- Radiation therapy is the primary treatment, with the standard approach involving 54–60 Gy over six weeks. Radiotherapy provides temporary improvement of symptoms and extends overall survival by an average of three months
- Numerous chemotherapy trials, both conventional and targeted, have been unsuccessful in improving survival, as these treatments were based largely on adult high-grade glioma strategies, which may not apply to DIPG due to its distinct biology

Further Reading

1. Grimm SA, Chamberlain MC. Brainstem glioma: a review. Curr Neurol Neurosci Rep 2013;13(5):346
2. Johung TB, Monje M. Diffuse intrinsic pontine glioma: new pathophysiological insights and emerging therapeutic targets. Curr Neuropharmacol 2017;15(1):88–97
3. Greenberg MS. Greenberg's Handbook of Neurosurgery. 10th ed. Stuttgart, Germany: Thieme Medical Publishing Group; 2023

Nitin Agarwal
David T. Fernandes Cabral
Samuel Adida

Thieme

Dural Arteriovenous Fistulas

15%

of all cerebral vascular malformations

- **The natural history of dAVFs with aggressive symptoms is poor, with annual rates of hemorrhage, CN deficits, and mortality at 7.4, 19.0, and 3.8%, respectively. Urgent treatment (endovascular, surgical, or combination) is recommended**
- **In contrast, dAVFs with benign symptoms, such as tinnitus or ophthalmologic issues, have better outcomes, with annual rates of hemorrhage, CN deficits, and mortality at 1.4, 1.5, and 0%, respectively**

PRESENTATION

- Dural arteriovenous fistulas (dAVFs) are vascular malformations in which arteries from the carotid or vertebral arteries drain into the dural venous sinuses; they termed carotid-cavernous fistulas when in the cavernous sinus
- Distinct from AVMs, dAVFs lack a parenchymal nidus and are supplied by vessels perfusing the dura. They commonly arise after dural sinus thrombosis, trauma, infection, or craniotomy, with 61–66% occurring in females
- Typically found at the transverse-sigmoid junction, cavernous sinus, superior sagittal sinus, anterior cranial fossa, and tentorium. Often diagnosed during evaluations for hemorrhage, seizures, CN palsies, focal deficits, or incidentally
- Pulsatile tinnitus is the most common presenting symptom; intracranial hemorrhage drives morbidity/mortality. Hemorrhage risk correlates with venous drainage patterns

RADIOGRAPHIC FEATURES

- MRA and CTA may demonstrate abnormal arteries and veins, sinus enlargement, or sinus occlusion. A six-vessel cerebral DSA is required to establish the diagnosis and plan treatment

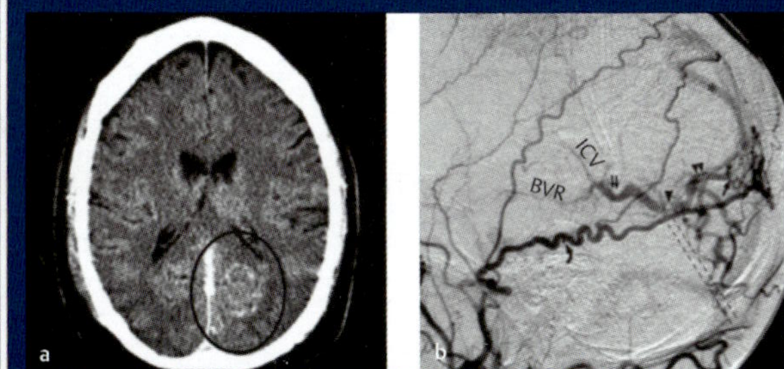

(a) CT with contrast showing engorged cortical veins; (b) CTA shows an enlarged middle meningeal artery (*curved arrow*), the fistulous point (*arrow*), posterior falcine sinus (*double arrowhead*), stenotic connection with straight sinus (*arrowhead*), stenosed straight sinus (*dashed lines*), retrograde flow into the vein of Galen (*double arrow*), further retrograde flow into the basal vein of Rosenthal (BVR), and internal cerebral veins (ICV)

TREATMENT

- The Borden and Cognard classification systems are used to describe the nature of intracranial daVFs. Spinal AVFs are classified differently

Borden classification		Cognard classification	
Type	Fistula location/venous drainage	Type	Fistula location/venous drainage
I	Venous sinus or meningeal vein(s)/antegrade in sinus(es) only	I	Venous sinus/antegrade in sinus(es)
		IIa	Venous sinus/retrograde in sinus(es)
II	Venous sinus or meningeal vein/retrograde in cortical vein(s)	IIb	Venous sinus/retrograde in cortical vein(s)
		IIa+b	Venous sinus/retrograde in both sinus(es) and cortical vein(s)
III	Cortical vein/retrograde in cortical vein(s)	III	Cortical vein (without venous ectasia)/retrograde in cortical vein(s)
		IV	Cortical vein (with venous ectasia)/retrograde in cortical vein(s)
		V	Cortical vein/retrograde in spinal perimedullary vein(s)

- For incidental cases, conservative management with monitoring is advised
- Treatment options in symptomatic patients include endovascular embolization, microsurgical disconnection, and SRS, with the goal of treatment to disconnect the fistula from its venous drainage. Tentorial and ethmoidal dAVMs are often treated surgically

Further Readings

1. Zyck S, Jesus O, Gould GC. Dural Arteriovenous Fistula. Treasure Island, FL: StatPearls Publishing; 2024
2. Reynolds MR, Lanzino G, Zipfel GJ. Intracranial dural arteriovenous fistulae. Stroke 2017;48(5):1424–1431
3. Greenberg MS. Greenberg's Handbook of Neurosurgery. 10th ed. New York, NY: Thieme Medical Publishing Group; 2023

Nitin Agarwal
David T. Fernandes Cabral
Samuel Adida

Thieme

Eosinophilic Granulomas

Eosinophilic granulomas often present with systemic conditions such as Letterer–Siwe or Hand–Schuller–Christian disease

Histopathology shows Langerhans cells with positivity for CD1 and S100, and electron microscopy shows Birbeck's granules

Single lesions of the skull are usually treated with excision and curettage. Lesions associated with systemic disease may be treated with chemotherapy and/or low-dose RT

ETIOLOGY

- Langerhans cell histiocytosis (LCH) is a rare, clonal proliferation of epidermal Langerhans cells, with eosinophilic granuloma as its mildest manifestation. Incidence is 4–5 cases per million annually in children under 15 years and 1–2 cases per million in adults, with a male predominance (1.2:1)
- Most commonly affects craniofacial bones (parietal and frontal), with intracranial involvement in the hypothalamic–pituitary axis (25–50%), meninges (30%), and choroid plexus (6%)
- Presents as tender, enlarging masses, often with pain and swelling. Single bone lesions account for 90% of cases, with 10% involving multiple bones or other organs (skin, pituitary gland, liver, spleen, lungs). They may also spontaneously regress
- LCH is associated with systemic symptoms including headache, increased thirst, and urination due to diabetes insipidus

RADIOGRAPHIC FEATURES

- X-ray reveals punched-out lytic bone lesions. CT shows bony destruction with central density. MRI typically shows hypointense to isointense lesions on T1, hyperintense lesions on T2 and STIR, and diffuse gadolinium enhancement on T1

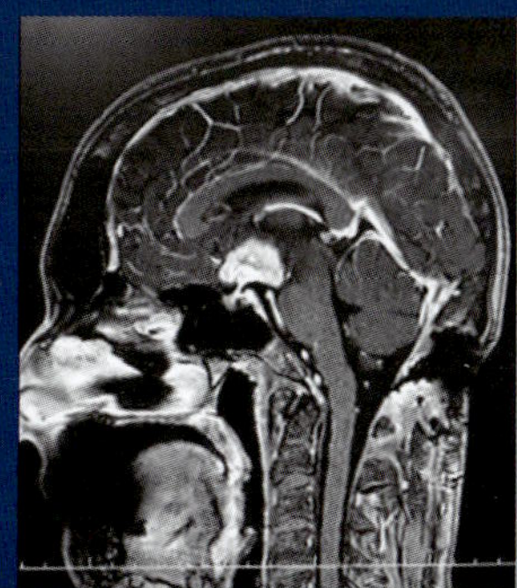

T1 MRI with contrast showing an eosinophilic granuloma in the hypothalamic–pituitary axis

OTHER CONSIDERATION

- Histopathology: Shows Langerhans cells with characteristic nuclear grooves ("coffee-bean" appearance), eosinophils, multinucleated Touton-like giant cells, inflammatory cells, and necrosis
- Immunohistochemistry: Positive for CD1, S100, CD207, and cyclin D1. BRAF VE1 mutations present in 50% of cases
- Electron microscopy: Reveals Birbeck's granules ("tennis racquet-shaped" inclusions)

TREATMENT

- Management: Symptomatic, persistent single skull lesions are treated with excision and curettage. Systemic disease or multiple lesions are managed with chemotherapy or low-dose radiation therapy
- Prognosis: Generally favorable, especially for patients with solitary lesions. Poorer prognosis is associated with high-risk features, such as multisystem involvement, skeletal maturity, multiple bone lesions, or skull base involvement

Further Readings

1. Greenberg MS. Greenberg's Handbook of Neurosurgery. 10h ed. New York, NY: Thieme Medical Publishing Group; 2023

Nitin Agarwal
David T. Fernandes Cabral
Samuel Adida

Thieme

Ependymal Tumors

2%
of all CNS tumors

- Clinical presentation:
  - Intracranial: Headache, nausea, vomiting, ataxia, CN deficits, and hydrocephalus
  - Spinal: Pain and motor or sensory deficits
- Treatment:
  - Gross total removal is the most important prognosticator of overall survival in both adults and children, and postoperative RT reduces recurrence

BACKGROUND

- Ependymal tumors are glial lesions originating from ependymal cells lining the ventricular system and are the third most common pediatric brain tumor. They have a bimodal distribution. Childhood cases typically present as posterior fossa ependymomas, while adult cases often involve spinal ependymomas
- Symptoms:
  - Intracranial ependymomas (especially posterior fossa): Headache, nausea, vomiting, ataxia, vertigo, CN deficits, hydrocephalus, and altered mental status such as confusion or lethargy
  - Spinal ependymomas: Pain and motor or sensory deficits
- Histopathology shows small, uniform cells with round nuclei that form pseudorosettes or ependymal rosettes within a fibrillary matrix
- Imaging:
  - Craniospinal axis imaging is essential due to the risk of drop metastases
  - MRI: Isointense to hypointense on T1, enhances on T1 with contrast, and hyperintense on T2
- Classification: Based on site, histology, and molecular biology features.

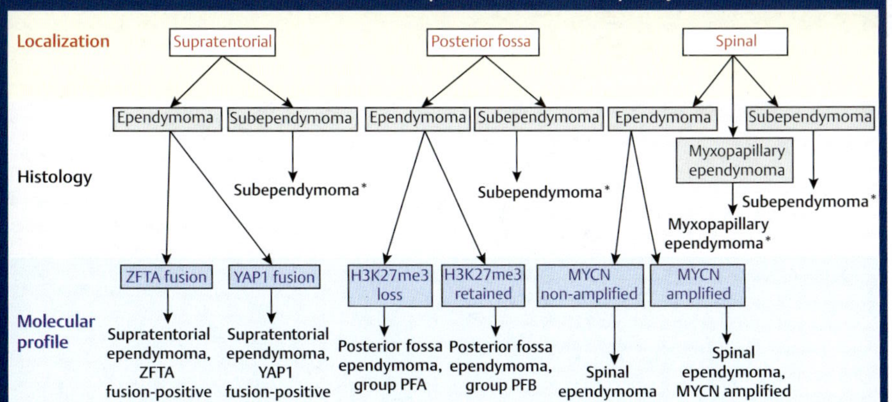

RADIOGRAPHIC FEATURES

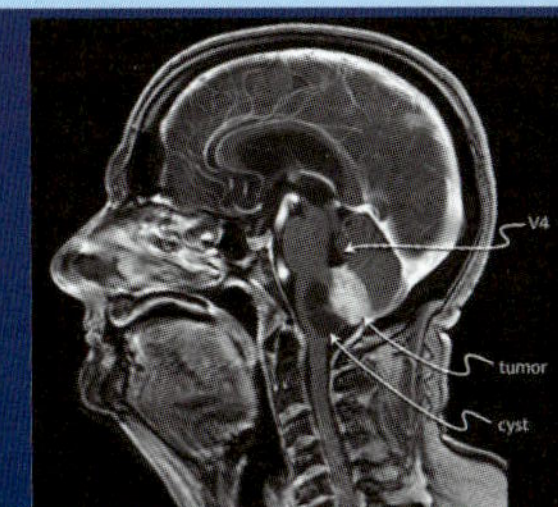

WHO grade II ependymoma arising from the 4th ventricle with a cystic component invading the medulla

TREATMENT

- Surgical outcomes: Complete resection without residual disease leads to better clinical outcomes and survival compared to partial resection
- Adjuvant RT: Improves survival and reduces the risk of local recurrence when used postoperatively
- Chemotherapy: Limited evidence supports its use in adult ependymoma

Further Readings
1. Zamora EA , Alkherayf F. Ependymoma. Treasure Island, FL: StatPearls Publishing; 2024
2. Greenberg MS. Greenberg's Handbook of Neurosurgery. 10th ed. New York, NY: Thieme Medical Publishing Group; 2023

Nitin Agarwal
David T. Fernandes Cabral
Samuel Adida

Thieme

Extracranial Carotid Artery Disease

Accounts for

15–20%

of all strokes

Influential clinical trials:

- NASCET: Demonstrated the benefit of CEA for symptomatic severe carotid stenosis (70 –99%)
- ECST: Showed CEA is beneficial for symptomatic carotid stenosis >70%
- CREST: Compared CEA and CAS, showing that CAS is non-inferior to CEA
- ACAS: Demonstrated CEA improves outcomes in asymptomatic carotid stenosis >60%
- SAPPHIRE: Proved CAS is safe and effective for high-risk patients
- CAVATAS: Showed that CAS is an alternative to CEA in high-risk symptomatic patients
- CREST-2: Ongoing trial comparing CEA and CAS in asymptomatic patients with carotid stenosis

ETIOLOGY

- Extracranial carotid artery disease (ECAD) is commonly caused by atherosclerotic plaque that forms on the CCA and extends into the lumen of the ICA
- The risk of stroke correlates with the degree of stenosis and atheroma morphology. It is also increased in hypercoagulable states

PRESENTATION

- Asymptomatic carotid artery disease is usually diagnosed following a routine physical examination and the detection of a carotid bruit
- Symptomatic cases are defined as focal neurological deficits due to TIA, amaurosis fugax, central retinal artery occlusion, or stroke attributable to the ICA with vessel narrowing. These symptoms should occur within six months of evaluation for therapy

IMAGING HALLMARKS

- Imaging choice depends on symptomatology. During the acute investigation of focal neurological deficit, a non-contrast CT and CTA may be performed for the evaluation of stroke or ischemia. For patients seen in the clinic with resolution of focal neurological deficits, MRI and MRA are typically used
- Carotid duplex ultrasound is typically ordered for those with an audible bruit who are considered asymptomatic. Patients with significant calcification of the carotid artery may be unsuitable for ultrasound
- Stenosis should be measured by comparing the ICA diameter at the most stenotic portion to the luminal diameter of the distal, disease-free extracranial ICA, with >50% stenosis per NASCET criteria using DSA, CTA, and/or MRA (both time-of-flight and contrast-enhanced MRI)
- Adequate evaluation of stenotic percentage generally requires two different imaging modalities that demonstrate concordance

TREATMENT

- Both asymptomatic and symptomatic ECAD require intensive medical management, including antithrombotic therapy, statins, and control of risk factors such as hypertension, smoking cessation, and diabetes mellitus
- Revascularization through CEA or carotid artery stenting for asymptomatic ECAD is common but often patient- and institution-specific, depending on atheroma morphology, patient life expectancy, and peri-procedural risk guidelines. Generally, CEA is considered for asymptomatic ECAD when stenosis is 70–99% and life expectancy is >5 years
- For symptomatic ECAD, CEA should be considered when stenosis is between 50 and 99%, as this range offers a greater potential for improved life expectancy, particularly when luminal narrowing is 70–99% compared to 50–70%. CEA is also preferred when revascularization is performed within 48 h to two weeks after symptom onset. While transfemoral CAS presents a higher peri-procedural risk of stroke and death compared to CEA, individual patient factors should be carefully evaluated when deciding between the two treatment options

Further Reading

1. Mohd AB, Alabdallat Y, Mohd OB et al. Medical and surgical management of symptomatic and asymptomatic carotid artery stenosis: a comprehensive literature review. Cureus 2023;15(8):e43263
2. Greenberg MS. Greenberg's Handbook of Neurosurgery. 10th ed. Stuttgart, Germany: Thieme Medical Publishing Group; 2023

Nitin Agarwal
David T. Fernandes Cabral
Samuel Adida

Thieme

Giant Cell Arteritis (GCA)

Demographics:
Caucasians
Age > 50; mean age: 70
Women > men

Late complications include blindness, stroke, thoracic aortic aneurysms, and aortic dissections

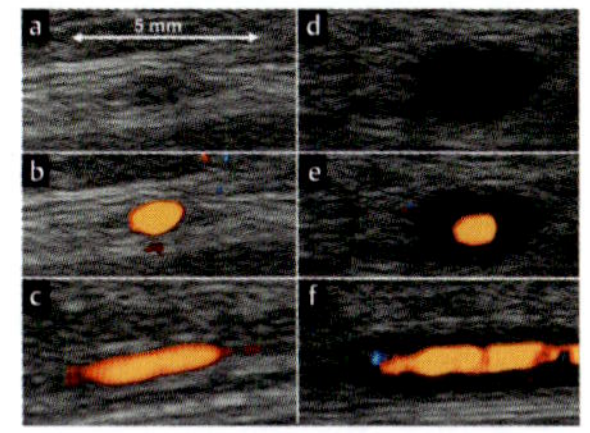

Duplex ultrasound of the superficial temporal artery. 22-MHz linear probe. (a–c) Normal individual. (d–f) GCA

OVERVIEW

- Pathophysiology: Granulomatous inflammation of arteries with infiltration predominantly by histiocytes, lymphocytes, and multinucleated giant cells (50% of cases)
    - Discontinuous ("skip-lesions") inflammatory response of lymphocytes, plasma cells, macrophages, ± giant cells affecting the media of arteries
- Typical arteries: Ophthalmic and posterior ciliary branches and entire external carotid system
    - Generally spares the renal artery
- Epidemiology: Most frequent form of vasculitis in persons older than 50 years; granulomatous chronic vasculitis involving large and medium-sized vessels, most commonly the temporal and other cranial arteries
- If left untreated, can lead to blindness
- Differential diagnosis:
    - Takayasu arteritis: Tends to affect large arteries in women; two phases, inflammatory and stenotic
- Temporal artery biopsy is recommended for all patients with suspected GCA

CLINICAL PRESENTATION

- Clinical presentation: Cranial neurological complications—temporal and occipital headache, visual loss, stroke, cognitive and psychiatric symptoms(dementia, depression, psychosis), cranial nerve impairment (oculomotor palsy, vestibular syndrome, jugular foramen syndrome); extracranial neurological complications—peripheral nerve neuropathy, radiculoplexopathy, mononeuropathy, myelopathy
- Headache: Most common presenting symptom
- Symptoms relating to ECA blood supply (jaw claudication, tongue, pharyngeal muscle)
- Ophthalmologic symptoms: Due to arteritis and occlusion of branches of the ophthalmic artery or posterior ciliary arteries
    - *Amaurosis fugax*, permanent blindness, vision field cuts, diplopia, ptosis, ocular pain, corneal edema, chemosis
- Temporal arteries may exhibit tenderness, swelling, erythema, pulsations
- Systemic symptoms: Fever, anorexia, weight loss, fatigue, malaise, neuropathy
    - The presence of systemic symptoms correlates with a *lower* incidence of blindness or stroke

MANAGEMENT

- Imaging modality: Ultrasonography, MRI, and FDG-PET
- Imaging hallmarks: Vascular imaging can fail to show arterial thickening or stenosis, so the identification of an "arterial halo" on ultrasound examination of the temporal artery is strongly suggestive of the diagnosis
- Laboratory studies:
    - ESR > 40
    - C-reactive protein
    - CBC: Mild normochromic anemia
    - Rheumatoid factor, ANA, serum complement usually normal
- Differential diagnosis:
    - Periarteritis nodosa (PAN)
    - Hypersensitivity vasculitis
- Temporal biopsy is optimally performed ahead of steroid treatment:
    - Sensitivity, 90% (range, 9–97%)
    - Specificity, near 100%
    - Predictive value, 94%
- Treatment:
    - Glucocorticoids (oral prednisone) are the cornerstone of remission induction in GCA, but targeted therapies can also be used to interfere with specific pathways
    - Tocilizumab

Nitin Agarwal
David T. Fernandes Cabral
Samuel Adida

Thieme

Glioblastomas (GBM)

Median survival after diagnosis is 14–16 months

Stupp protocol

- **Initial treatment:**
  - **RT: 60 Gy (in 30 fractions) over 6 weeks**
  - **TMZ: 75 mg/m² per day orally, administered concurrently with RT (on days 1–42)**
- **Adjuvant treatment:**
  - **After completing RT, TMZ is continued at 150–200 mg/m² orally, on days 1–5 of a 28-day cycle for 6 cycles**

PRESENTATION

- Glioblastoma (GBM) is the most malignant and pervasive glioma subtype (WHO grade 4) and the most common primary brain tumor in adults
- Nearly 90% of GBMs are IDH wild type, arising de novo. The only established risk factor is high-dose ionizing radiation
- Early symptoms include headaches, seizures, and focal neurological deficits, with general symptoms such as nausea, vomiting, cognitive difficulties, personality changes, and gait disorders. Seizures occur in 20% of cases, with an additional 20% developing them later
- GBM commonly affects the frontal or temporal lobes. MRI typically reveals large, irregular ring-enhancing lesions with a central necrotic core, which may or may not contain hemorrhage, surrounded by vasogenic edema; approximately 20% of cases are multifocal
- The histopathological hallmarks of GBM include high mitotic activity, pseudopalisading necrosis, and microvascular proliferation

RADIOGRAPHIC FEATURES

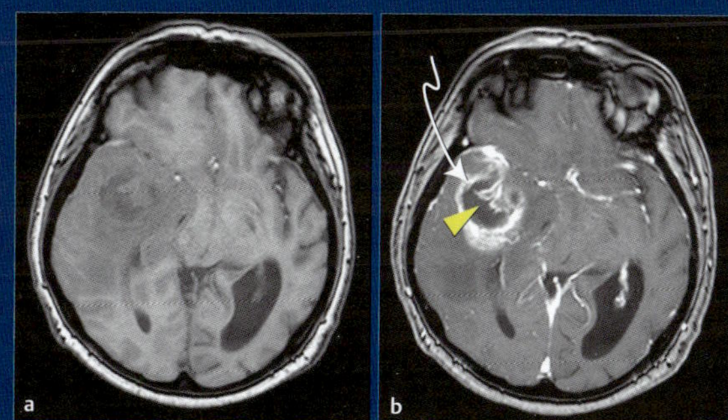

(a) T1 noncontrast and (b) with contrast MRI of an IDH wild-type temporal lobe GBM. Of note, the characteristic area of central necrosis is indicated by the *yellow arrowhead*

OTHER CONSIDERATIONS

- Molecular characteristics include wild-type status with no mutations in IDH1/IDH2, TERT promoter mutations, EGFR gene amplification, and chromosome 7p gain and 10q loss; CDKN2A/CDKN2B deletions may also be present

TREATMENT

- Treatment involves maximal safe surgical resection followed by adjuvant RT and temozolomide (TMZ) as per the Stupp protocol. The modified Stupp protocol is utilized in elderly patients. Resection allows for cytoreduction and histological diagnosis
- Side effects of TMZ include nausea, vomiting, fatigue, headache, constipation, loss of appetite, bone marrow suppression, and seizures
- RT for small lesions or recurrent lesions subject to reirradiation includes laser interstitial RT, SRS, whole-brain RT, and proton beam therapy

Further Readings

1. Kanderi T, Munakomi S, Gupta V. Glioblastoma Multiforme. Treasure Island, FL: StatPearls Publishing; 2024
2. Perry JR, Laperriere N, O'Callaghan CJ, et al. Short-course radiation plus temozolomide in elderly patients with glioblastoma. N Engl J Med 2017;376(11):1027–1037
3. Greenberg MS. Greenberg's Handbook of Neurosurgery. 10th ed. New York, NY: Thieme Medical Publishing Group; 2023

Nitin Agarwal
David T. Fernandes Cabral
Samuel Adida

Thieme

Hemangioblastomas (HB)

- 75–80% of lesions are sporadic
- Peak age of sporadic hemangioblastoma is 30–60 years

Genetics:

- von Hippel-Lindau (VHL) syndrome
- Chromosome 3
- Autosomal dominant

Most common locations:

- Cerebellum: 45–65%
- Spinal cord: 3–36%
- Cauda equina: 11%
- Brainstem: 5%
- Supratentorial: 1% (VHL patients)

PRESENTATION

- Capillary hemangiomas
- Most common primary intra-axial posterior fossa tumor in adults
- Most commonly in the cerebellum, spinal cord, medulla
- Symptoms:
  - Headaches
  - Hydrocephalus
  - Cerebellar dysfunction
  - Altered mental state
  - Polycythemia due to erythropoietin production

PATHOLOGY

- WHO Grade I (benign)
- Juvenile: thin-walled capillaries and dilated vessels tightly packed
- Transitional: thin-walled capillaries and dilated vessels intermingled with stromal cells
- Clear cell: sheets of xanthoma cells

RADIOGRAPHIC FEATURES

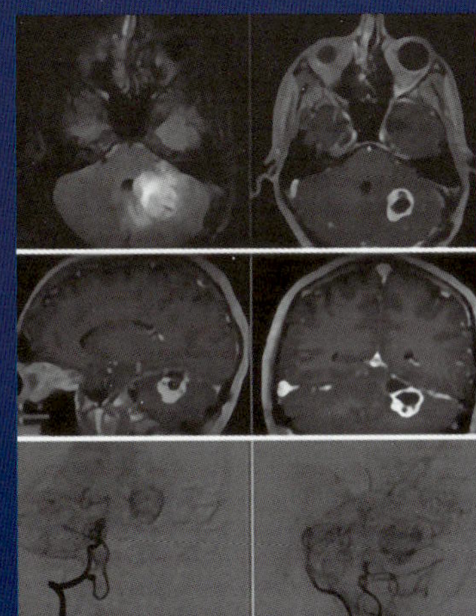

- Vertebral artery angiography will demonstrate intense vascularity
- T1 MRI: Isointense mural nodule
- T2 MRI: Hyperintense mural nodule, flow voids
- CT: Isodense mural nodule, postcontrast intense homogeneous enhancement

EVALUATION/TREATMENT

- Evaluation
  - CT
  - MRI: contrast enhancing nodule
  - +/− Angiography
  - Labs
    - May reveal polycythemia
    - Rule out catecholamine production
- Further imaging/examination (renal lesions, intraocular lesions, etc.) in setting of VHL
- Surgical resection +/− embolization may be curative in sporadic HGB
  - Cyst wall not neoplastic, can be left behind (as compared to pilocytic)
- Radiation treatment may reduce tumor size/prevent growth

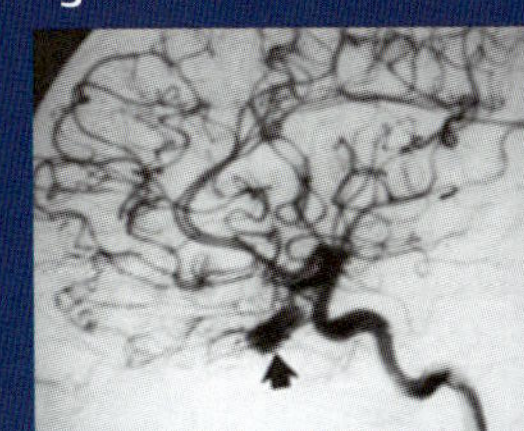

Further Reading

1. Panigrahi M, Schirmer C, Singh L, eds. Neurosurgery Updates: Controversies in Vascular Surgery. 1st ed. Noida: Thieme; 2021: Volume 2
2. Spetzler RF, Kalani MYS, Nakaji P, Yagmurlu K. Color Atlas of Brainstem Surgery. Noida: Thieme; 2021.

Nitin Agarwal
David T. Fernandes Cabral
Regan Shanahan

Thieme

Hemifacial Spasm (HFS)

Hemifacial spasm occurs most frequently in women over the age of 40, with a prevalence ratio of 2:1 compared to men

The typical presentation includes unilateral, intermittent, painless, involuntary spasms of the muscles innervated by the facial (VII) nerve

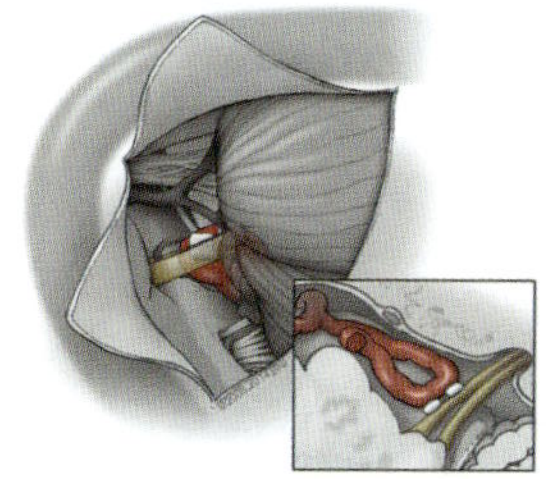

The most common offending vessel is the AICA

DESCRIPTION

- Begins with contractions of orbicularis oculi and progresses to the entire half of the face
- Persists during sleep
- Atypical presentation with buccal muscle involvement is more resistant to treatment
- Associated symptoms of vestibulocochlear (VIII) compression:
  - Vertigo
  - Tinnitus
  - Hearing loss
- Differential diagnosis:
  - Blepharospasm
    - Typically, only involves the orbicularis oculi, whereas hemifacial spasm can involve all parts of the face
  - Facial myokymia
    - Rare disorder that causes involuntary, continuous, and rippling movements of the facial muscles

ETIOLOGY/DIAGNOSIS

- Compression of the facial nerve at the root exit zone (REZ) that typically impinges the anterocaudal aspect of VII/VIII nerve complex

- Hemifacial spasm can arise from:
  - Vascular compression syndrome (most common)
  - Idiopathic
  - Tumor compressing the nerve
  - Post bell's palsy

<u>Babinksi-2 sign</u>: Lifting of the ipsilateral eyebrow with eye closure during the spasm is highly specific and sensitive for the condition.

<u>Lateral spread test:</u> Electrophysiological test that detects an "abnormal muscle response" called the "lateral spread response (LSR)" during electromyography (EMG), where stimulation of one branch of the facial nerve causes unintended muscle contractions in other facial muscle branches

EVALUATION/TREATMENT

- Typically, a diagnosis of omission (rule out: tumor and AVM)
- Medical management options:
  - Carbamazepine
  - Phenytoin
  - Botox injections, q3–6 months
- Surgical management: Microvascular decompression
- 10% recurrence rate
- Complications
  - Total hearing loss
  - Partial hearing loss
  - Transient facial weakness
  - Permanent facial weakness
  - Ataxia

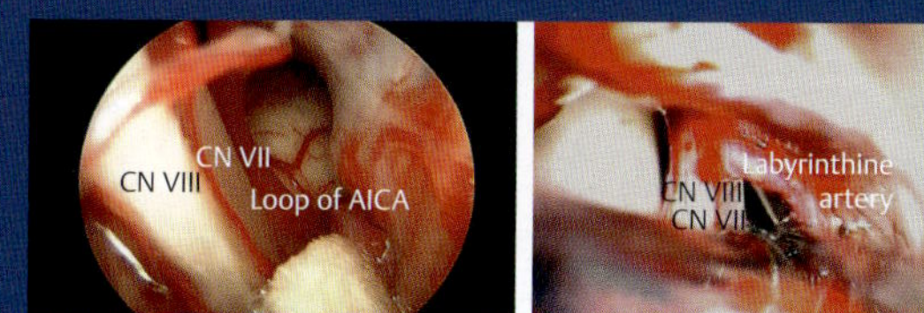

Further Readings

1. Wei X, Wang J, Kong X, Gao C, Wang F. Effect of microvascular decompression of the vagus root entry/exit zone on blood pressure in patients with hemifacial spasm associated with essential hypertension: a retrospective clinical analysis. J Neurol Surg B Skull Base 2022;83(S02):336–342
2. Nakaji P, Zaidi HA, eds. Controversies in Neuroendoscopy. 1st ed. New York: Thieme; 2019

Nitin Agarwal
David T. Fernandes Cabral
Regan Shanahan

Thieme

Overview of Hemorrhagic Stroke-Part I

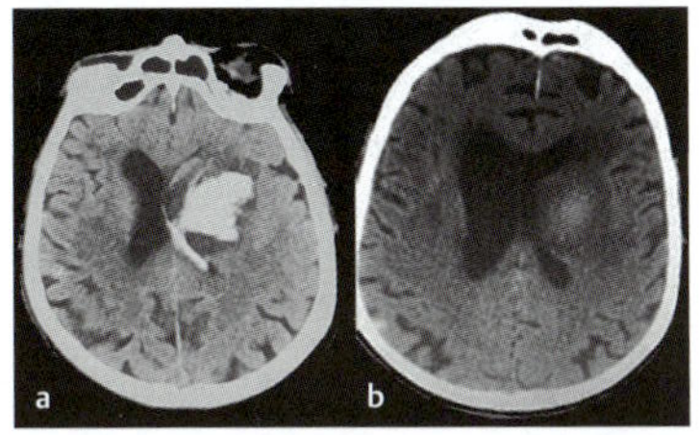

(a) A noncontrast head computed tomography (CT) shows an acute deep cerebral hemorrhage in the left basal ganglia with surrounding vasogenic edema, followed by an intraventricular hemorrhage with no midsagittal plane shift. (b) The follow-up CT scan showed significant resorption of the basal ganglia hematoma

OVERVIEW

Introduction

- Hemorrhagic stroke refers to bleeding within the brain and is primarily classified into intracerebral hemorrhage (ICH) and subarachnoid hemorrhage (SAH). These types of strokes are associated with a high rate of morbidity and mortality, especially in cases of ICH, where prompt recognition and management are essential to prevent secondary brain injury. Hemorrhagic strokes can occur spontaneously or secondary to trauma, vascular malformations, or aneurysms

Etiology

ICH

- Occurs when a cerebral artery or arteriole ruptures, leading to blood leakage into the brain parenchyma. This results in direct parenchymal injury, increased intracranial pressure (ICP), and brain compression
- Common causes:
    - Hypertension (chronic) leads to microaneurysms and arteriolar wall rupture
    - Cerebral amyloid angiopathy (CAA), which occurs in elderly patients, weakens vessel walls
    - Coagulopathy, either from medications (e.g., anticoagulants) or clotting disorders
    - Vascular malformations such as arteriovenous malformations (AVMs) or cavernous malformations
    - Brain tumors (tumor-related hemorrhage) and infections
- Pathophysiology: Hemorrhage within the brain parenchyma can compress adjacent structures, disrupt normal brain function, and increase ICP, which may lead to herniation and death if not managed promptly

SAH

- Refers to bleeding into the subarachnoid space, typically from a ruptured aneurysm, most commonly in the anterior circulation (circle of Willis), especially at the anterior communicating artery or posterior communicating artery.
- Causes include the following:
    - Ruptured aneurysms (primary cause in 85% of nontraumatic SAH)
    - AVMs or cavernous malformations
    - Trauma (e.g., head injury causing direct blood vessel rupture)
- Pathophysiology: Blood in the subarachnoid space can obstruct cerebrospinal fluid (CSF) flow, leading to hydrocephalus, and cause vasospasm, which can result in ischemic brain injury. Rebleeding is a serious concern in the early hours postrupture

Further Readings

1. Radovic M, Micovic M, Zivkovic B, Bascarevic V. A strike from the air: cerebral hemorrhage after a lightning strike. Indian J Neurosurg 2024 (e-pub ahead of print). doi:10.1055/s-0044-1790534
2. Neto S, Flores JC, Figueiredo EG, Caldas JG, Teixeira MJ. Mycotic aneurysm treated with aneurysm trapping. Case report. J Neurol Surg Rep 2016;77(01):013–016
3. Gaillard F, Campos A, Sharma R, et al. Intracranial hemorrhage. Radiopaedia.org. Accessed March 20, 2025 at: https://radiopaedia.org/articles/intracranial-haemorrhage

Nitin Agarwal
David T. Fernandes Cabral
Regan Shanahan

Thieme

Overview of Hemorrhagic Stroke-Part II

Hunt and Hess Score for SAH

- **Grade 1: Asymptomatic or mild headache; no neurological deficits. Good prognosis**
- **Grade 2: Moderate headache and nuchal rigidity (neck stiffness); no or mild neurological deficits. Fair prognosis**
- **Grade 3: Drowsy or confused; mild focal neurological deficits (e.g., hemiparesis). Guarded prognosis**
- **Grade 4: Stuporous with severe focal neurological deficits, hemiplegia, or other signs of significant brain injury. Poor prognosis.**
- **Grade 5: Comatose, posturing, or severe neurological impairment (e.g., decerebrate rigidity). Very poor prognosis**

OVERVIEW

ICH

- Acute onset of focal neurological deficits: Hemiparesis, dysphagia, aphasia, or visual changes depending on the location of the bleed
- Headache is often severe and associated with nausea and vomiting
- Rapid progression: Patients may become drowsy, confused, or comatose as ICP increases
- Signs of increased ICP: Cushing's reflex, papilledema, and decreased level of consciousness
- Severe cases may present with seizures or signs of brain herniation

SAH

- Sudden onset of a severe headache, often described as the "worst headache of life."
- Neck stiffness (due to irritation of the meninges), nausea, and vomiting
- Loss of consciousness may occur, ranging from brief syncope to coma
- Focal neurological deficits may occur depending on the presence of associated complications (e.g., hydrocephalus, vasospasm, or rebleeding)
- Seizures may be seen in both ICH and SAH

Imaging

- Noncontrast CT is the first-line imaging modality for identifying ICH and SAH. It will show hyperdense areas in the brain parenchyma (for ICH) and hyperdense blood in the subarachnoid space (for SAH)
- CT angiography (CTA) may be used to identify the source of hemorrhage, particularly in SAH cases to locate ruptured aneurysms
- MRI is not typically used for the acute diagnosis of hemorrhage but is helpful in assessing the extent of damage, particularly in ICH for evaluating surrounding edema or ischemia
    - MR angiography (MRA) can be used for detecting aneurysms or AVMs in the setting of SAH
- Lumbar puncture (LP; for SAH diagnosis when CT is negative):
    - Xanthochromia (yellow-tinged CSF) is a key finding in SAH, indicating the presence of old blood
    - Elevated opening pressure can also be indicative of increased ICP

Nitin Agarwal
David T. Fernandes Cabral
Regan Shanahan

Thieme

Overview of Hemorrhagic Stroke-Part III

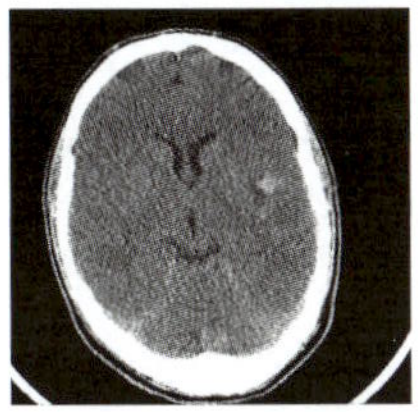

CT of the head with Fisher IV SAH

Fisher Grading for SAH

- Grade 1: No blood or minimal blood in the subarachnoid space
  - Low risk of vasospasm
- Grade 2: Blood in the subarachnoid space, but no significant amounts in the basal cisterns or ventricles
  - Moderate risk of vasospasm
- Grade 3: Blood present in the basal cisterns or ventricles, or significant clot formation
  - High risk of vasospasm
- Grade 4: Diffuse blood throughout the subarachnoid space with extensive clot formation and/or intraventricular hemorrhage
  - Very high risk of vasospasm, as well as poorer clinical outcomes

MANAGEMENT

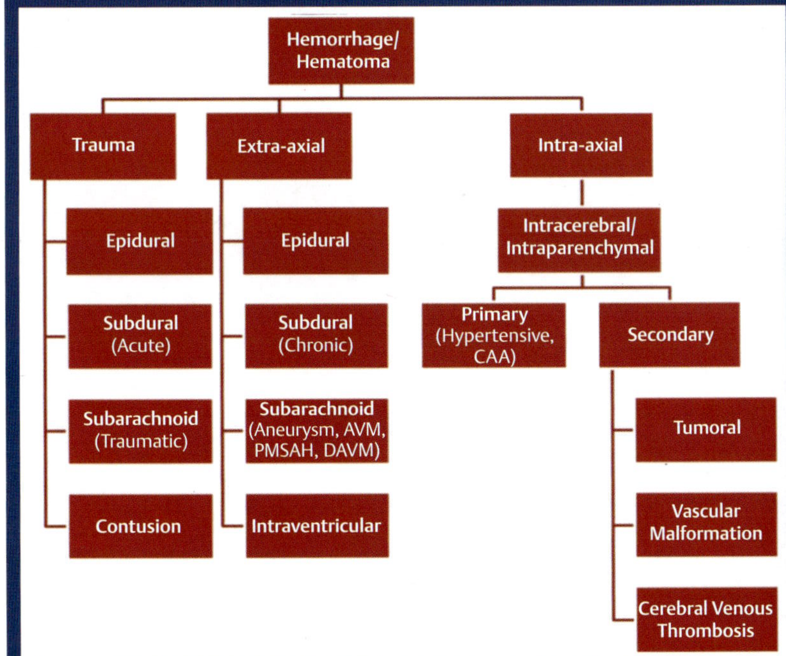

Prognosis

- ICH prognosis is generally poor, especially in the presence of large hematomas, midline shift, or severe ICP increase. Early surgical intervention and aggressive management improve outcomes
- SAH prognosis depends on the Hunt and Hess grade, with higher grades correlating with worse outcomes. Prompt aneurysm repair and prevention of rebleeding are key to improving survival
- Rehabilitation plays a crucial role in improving functional recovery poststroke

Nitin Agarwal
David T. Fernandes Cabral
Regan Shanahan

Thieme

Ventriculoperitoneal (VP) Shunt-Part I

VP shunt placement is the gold standard treatment for hydrocephalus, diverting CSF from the ventricles to the peritoneal cavity. The procedure involves careful surgical placement of the ventricular catheter, valve, and distal catheter, often requiring ongoing monitoring for function and complications

ETIOLOGY

- A ventriculoperitoneal (VP) shunt is a surgical device used to treat hydrocephalus (excess cerebrospinal fluid [CSF] within the brain)
- The shunt provides a way to divert CSF from the ventricular system of the brain to the peritoneal cavity (abdominal area), where the fluid can be absorbed
- The VP shunt is one of the most common procedures performed in neurosurgery, especially for pediatric and adult patients with hydrocephalus

Indications

- Obstructive hydrocephalus: Caused by a blockage of the CSF pathways, such as from tumors, cysts, or aqueductal stenosis
- Communicating hydrocephalus: Caused by impaired absorption of CSF, such as in normal pressure hydrocephalus (NPH) or due to meningeal fibrosis
- Congenital hydrocephalus: Conditions like aqueductal stenosis, Chiari malformations, or Dandy–Walker malformations often present with congenital hydrocephalus, which may require shunting
- Postsurgical hydrocephalus: Following neurosurgical procedures, such as tumor resection, cranial surgery, or hemorrhages, some patients may develop hydrocephalus
- Traumatic brain injury (TBI): Hydrocephalus can develop after significant head trauma, leading to increased ICP and the need for a VP shunt
- Infections (e.g., meningitis or ventriculitis) causing CSF flow obstruction or impaired absorption may require shunting as a secondary intervention

Further Reading

1. Shah A, Singh D, Loomba P, Singh H, Mittal A, Srivastava S. Peroral extrusion of ventriculoperitoneal shunt: an unusual complication and review of literature. Indian J Neurosurg 2016;05(03):196–201

Nitin Agarwal
David T. Fernandes Cabral
Regan Shanahan

Thieme

Ventriculoperitoneal (VP) Shunt-Part II

Postoperative monitoring is critical to identify complications like shunt malfunction (blockage or dislodgement), infection, and over- or under-drainage. Timely recognition and intervention are crucial for preventing further neurological damage or infection

PROCEDURE

Components of a VP Shunt

A VP shunt system typically consists of the following components:

- Ventricular catheter: Inserted into the lateral ventricle or third ventricle to drain excess CSF
- Valve: Regulates the flow of CSF from the ventricles to the peritoneal cavity

Different types of valves can be used, such as the following:

- Fixed-pressure valves: Open when CSF pressure exceeds a certain threshold
- Adjustable valves: Allow for postoperative adjustment of CSF drainage pressure
- Distal catheter: Runs from the valve and is placed in the peritoneal cavity, typically in the abdomen. CSF is then absorbed into the peritoneal lining
- Pump (optional): Some shunts incorporate a pump or an external reservoir for adjusting or monitoring pressure

Surgical Technique

- Preoperative planning: Preoperative imaging (usually CT or MRI) to assess the ventricular size and anatomy, as well as the presence of any possible obstructions to CSF flow
- Incision and exposure: The procedure typically involves two incisions, one on the scalp to insert the ventricular catheter and one in the abdominal area for the distal catheter placement
- Burr hole is drilled over the parietal lobe to access the lateral ventricle. The ventricular catheter is then inserted
- Catheter placement: The ventricular catheter is advanced into the lateral ventricle or third ventricle. In cases of obstructive hydrocephalus, care is taken to avoid damaging any structures that could worsen the obstruction
    - The distal catheter is tunneled under the skin to the peritoneal cavity (pressure is near atmospheric), where it is inserted into the abdomen. Some other types of shunts may involve the right atrium or pleural space depending on anatomy
- Valve and final adjustment: The valve is connected between the ventricular catheter and the distal catheter. The valve regulates the amount of CSF that drains based on pressure
- The system is tested intraoperatively for functionality, ensuring proper drainage and no signs of obstruction
- Wound closure: Both scalp and abdominal incisions are closed with sutures or staples. Postoperative monitoring focuses on drainage and signs of infection or complications

Nitin Agarwal
David T. Fernandes Cabral
Regan Shanahan

Thieme

Ventriculoperitoneal (VP) Shunt-Part III

Inguinal hernia occurs in 17% of cases in which the shunt is inserted when the processus vaginalis is patent

COMPLICATIONS

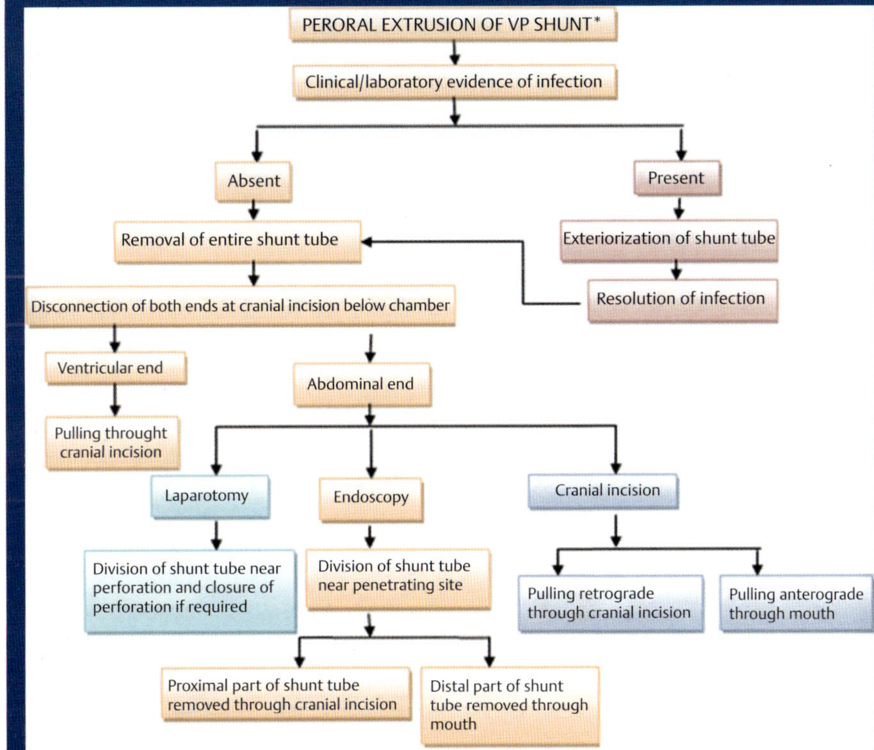

* If hydrocephalus is present, a new VP shunt needs to be placed.

indicates treatment used in our case.

Complications

- Shunt malfunction: Shunt blockage or dislodgement can lead to failure to drain CSF, resulting in hydrocephalus. Symptoms include headache, vomiting, and increased intracranial pressure (ICP)
    - Over-drainage can occur, leading to subdural hematomas or cerebral herniation due to excessive CSF removal
- Infection: Infection at the insertion site or in the shunt system can occur, resulting in fever, redness, or pus drainage. The most common organisms are *Staphylococcus aureus* and coagulase-negative staphylococci
    - Meningitis is a serious complication and may require antibiotic therapy and shunt removal in severe cases
- Abdominal complications: The distal catheter placed in the peritoneum can lead to issues like peritonitis, bowel perforation, or hernia
    - Ascites or pseudocyst formation in the abdomen may occur in rare cases
- Shunt migration: The shunt can migrate out of its intended position, causing obstruction or ineffective drainage, requiring revision surgery. Migration may occur into the scrotum, viscus, stomach, bladder, etc.
- Over- or under-drainage: Over-drainage (more likely than ventriculoatrial shunt) can result in the collapse of ventricles and subdural hematomas, while under-drainage can lead to continued hydrocephalus symptoms. Proper valve adjustments may be needed to correct these issues

Nitin Agarwal
David T. Fernandes Cabral
Regan Shanahan

Thieme

Hydrocephalus and Cerebrospinal Fluid (CSF) Disorders

Workup:
- **Neurological examination and neuroimaging are performed to identify potential causes of obstruction and sites for shunt access**
- **Lumbar puncture or ICP monitoring is used to evaluate CSF dynamics and pressure**

PRESENTATION

- Hydrocephalus is a condition characterized by a disruption in the production, flow, or absorption of CSF. It can be idiopathic or secondary to various causes, including hemorrhage, tumors, infections, vascular lesions, surgery, or neurodegenerative diseases such as dementia
- Symptoms arise from increased ICP and may include headache, nausea, vomiting, gait abnormalities, imbalance, fatigue, incontinence, impaired vision, cognitive decline, memory loss, and dementia
- Radiographic features, including sulcal effacement, may be unreliable, as they can be similar to the features observed in hydrocephalus ex vacuo. Transependymal flow is more indicative of hydrocephalus

Enlarged ventricles

- Communicating
  - No obstruction to absorption of CSF
    - **Special types**
      This group is dominated my a miscellaneous collection of conditions which complex, and often poorly understood CSF dynamics.
      Examples include:
      - Choroid plexus papilloma*
      - NPH**
      Other causes of enlarged ventricles with normal probably normal CSF dynamics also fall into this category, although usually we do not refer to them as hydrocephalus. Examples include:
      - Hydrocephalus ex vacuo
      - Colpocephalus
  - Absorption of CSF obstructed
    - **Communicating hydrocephalus**
      This group is characterised by a process which obliterates or damages the normal arachnoid granulations, or prevents normal flow of CSF over the surface of the brain.
      Common causes include:
      - SAH (acute and chronic)
      - Meningitis
      - Bacterial
      - TB
      - Leptomeningeal carcinomatosis
- Non-communicating
  - Obstruction to normal absorption of CSF thus always present
    - **Obstructive hydrocephalus**
      This group is characterised by mechanical impedance to CSF leaving the ventricular system.
      Common causes include:
      - Masses compressing the ventricular system at any level (e.g. tectal plate glioma, colloid cyst, posterior fossa mass etc..)
      - Congenital aqueduct stenosis

**Choroid plexus papillomas are classically thought of as resulting in hydrocephalus by excessive production of CSF, although debris from the tumour is also believed to cause impaired obstruction to CSF absorption at the level of the arachnoid villi. In many instances the mass may also result in an obstructive component.
**Normal pressure hydrocephalus (NPH) is a controversial entity the cause of which remains incompletely understood, and abnormal CSF dynamics are thought to play a role

Management:
- **Acetazolamide, used to reduce CSF production, may cause hypokalemia**
- **Serial ventricular taps or lumbar punctures for symptomatic relief**
- **Definitive treatment depends on the underlying cause and may include endoscopic third ventriculostomy, obstruction removal, choroid plexectomy, and shunting**

ACCESS POINTS

Frazier's Point	Dandy's Point	Keen's Point
3 cm lateral to midline 6 cm superior to inion Trajectory: Toward contralateral medial canthus, ependyma should be reached at 4 cm. Soft passed to 8 cm	2 cm lateral to midline 3 cm superior to inion Trajectory: Perpendicular to skull, slightly superior, ependyma reached at 4 cm Soft passed to 8 cm	3 cm superior to pinna 3 cm posterior to pinna Trajectory: Perpendicular to skull, ependyma reached at 4 cm Soft passed to 8 cm

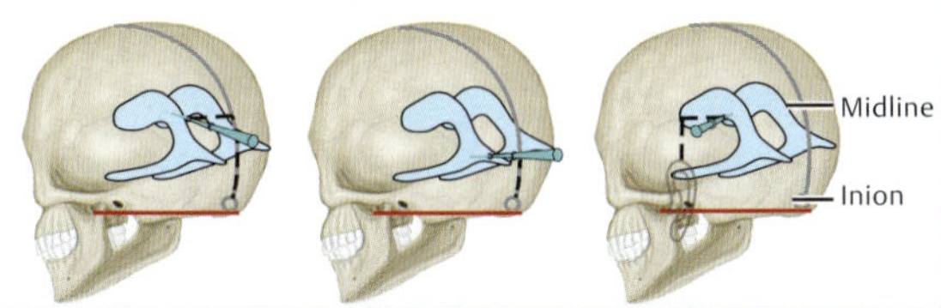

ABSORPTION POINTS

- **Ventriculo-peritoneal, ventriculo-atrial, ventriculo-pleural, ventriculo-cisternal (Torkildsen), ventriculo-subgaleal, ventriculo-subcutaneous, ventriculo-gallbladder, and ventriculo-iliac crest**

Nitin Agarwal
David T. Fernandes Cabral
Samuel Adida

Further Reading
1. Bir SC, Patra DP, Maiti TK et al. Epidemiology of adult-onset hydrocephalus: institutional experience with 2001 patients. Neurosurg Focus 2016;41(3):E5
2. Greenberg MS. Greenberg's Handbook of Neurosurgery. 10th ed. Stuttgart, Germany: Thieme Medical Publishing Group; 2023
3. Munakomi S, Das JM. Ventriculostomy. In: StatPearls [Internet]. Treasure Island, FL: StatPearls Publishing;2024

IDH-Mutant Gliomas

- **Oligodendrogliomas (IDH-mutant, 1p/19q codeleted) generally confer a more favorable prognosis**
- **Astrocytomas (IDH-mutant, ATRX/TP53-mutated) typically carry a worse prognosis, particularly if CDKN2A/B deletion is present**

- **Maximal safe resection improves survival and allows for molecular analysis:**
  - **Adjuvant therapy:**
    - **WHO grade 2: Surveillance for low-risk patients (age < 40, GTR), and RT with chemotherapy (PCV/TMZ) for high-risk patients (age > 40, subtotal resection)**
    - **WHO grade 3: RT with chemotherapy (PCV/TMZ)**

BACKGROUND

- IDH mutation and 1p/19q codeletion status are important prognostic markers for glioma. IDH mutations are present in over 80% of WHO grade 2 and 3 gliomas. In grade 4 GBM, IDH mutations are more common in secondary GBM (73%) compared to primary GBM (4%)
- The presence of IDH mutations is associated with improved outcomes, with longer survival in both GBM (IDH-wild-type: 15 months, IDH-mutant: 31 months) and anaplastic astrocytoma (IDH-wild-type: 20 months, IDH-mutant: 65 months)
- The high frequency of IDH mutations in secondary GBM suggests that low-grade gliomas with IDH mutations often undergo malignant transformation. IDH-mutated gliomas are also prone to developing a hypermutation phenotype, correlating with worse prognoses

RADIOGRAPHIC FEATURES

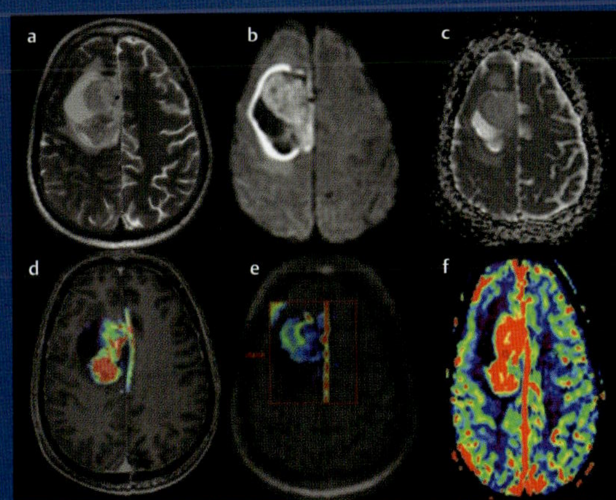

(a) T2, (b) DWI, (c) ADC, and (d–f) dynamic contrast-enhanced MRI of an IDH-mutant astrocytoma in the right superior frontal gyrus

TREATMENT

- Standard care for IDH-mutant glioma includes surgery, RT, and chemotherapy. Treatment starts with maximal safe resection to reduce symptoms and enable molecular analysis. The extent of resection is linked to better survival
- For grade 2 IDH-mutant gliomas, low-risk patients (age ≤ 40, gross total resection) may undergo a "watch-and-wait" approach, while high-risk patients (age > 40, subtotal resection) typically receive RT and chemotherapy with procarbazine, lomustine, and vincristine (PCV) or temozolomide (TMZ). The recent INDIGO trial showed that vorasidenib, an IDH1/2 inhibitor, significantly improves survival
- For grade 3 IDH-mutant gliomas, all patients receive RT followed by TMZ or PCV. The choice depends on 1p/19q status, with codeletion favoring PCV
- Ongoing trials (POLCA, NOA-18) are exploring chemotherapy alone as an upfront treatment. Salvage therapy after progression typically involves surgery, RT, and alkylating chemotherapy

Further Reading

1. Han S, Liu Y, Cai SJ et al. IDH mutation in glioma: molecular mechanisms and potential therapeutic targets. Br J Cancer 2020;122:1580–1589
2. Lin MD, Tsai AC, Abdullah KG, McBrayer SK, Shi DD. Treatment of IDH-mutant glioma in the INDIGO era. NPJ Precis Oncol 2024;8(1):149
3. Greenberg MS. Greenberg's Handbook of Neurosurgery. 10th ed. Stuttgart, Germany: Thieme Medical Publishing Group; 2023

Samuel Adida

Thieme

IDH-Wild-Type Gliomas

IDH-wild-type gliomas are generally associated with poor outcomes, especially when characterized by EGFR amplification, CDKN2A/B deletions, or 7+/10– chromosomal alterations

Stupp protocol:
- **Initial treatment:**
  - **RT: 60 Gy (in 30 fractions) over six weeks**
  - **TMZ: 75 mg/m² per day orally, administered concurrently with RT (on day 1 through 42)**
- **Adjuvant treatment:**
  - **After completing RT, TMZ is continued at 150–200 mg/m² orally, on days 1–5 of a 28-day cycle for six cycles**

BACKGROUND

- Adult-type diffuse gliomas make up over 90% of gliomas and include three main types: IDH-mutant astrocytoma, IDH-mutant and 1p/19q-codeleted oligodendroglioma, and IDH-wild-type GBM. Other glioma subtypes are rarer and tend to affect children, adolescents, and young adults, with lower-grade gliomas being the most common brain tumors in children
- Advancements in understanding glioma molecular pathogenesis have led to new tumor classifications, particularly in children, and improved diagnostic precision through molecular biomarkers and DNA methylation profiles
- While the treatment of WHO grade 2 and 3 gliomas has improved with the use of chemotherapy and RT based on molecular markers, treatment options for WHO grade 4 gliomas, particularly IDH-wild-type GBM, remain limited

RADIOGRAPHIC FEATURES

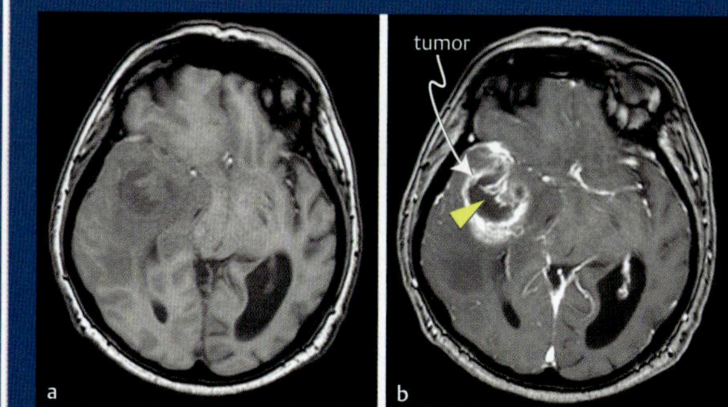

MRI with and without contrast of an IDH-wild-type GBM in the right temporal lobe

TREATMENT

- Maximal safe surgical resection improves survival. The Stupp protocol has become the standard of care following resection, administering temozolomide (TMZ) as follows:
  - Initial treatment:
    - RT: 60 Gy (in 30 fractions) over six weeks
    - TMZ: 75 mg/m² per day orally, administered concurrently with RT (on day 1 through 42)
  - Adjuvant treatment:
    - After completing RT, TMZ is continued at 150–200 mg/m² orally, on days 1–5 of a 28-day cycle for six cycles
- Improves survival from 12.1 months with RT alone to 14.6 months with the addition of TMZ
- Modified Stupp protocol:
  - Tumor-treating fields: Added during adjuvant phase, improved survival (20.9 months)
  - Short-course radiation: 40–45 Gy (in 15 fractions) for elderly or frail patients
  - Dose-dense temozolomide: Higher and more frequent dosing schedules
  - Immunotherapy: Use of checkpoint inhibitors such as nivolumab or pembrolizumab
  - Bevacizumab: For edema or recurrent GBM

Further Reading

1. Weller M, Wen PY, Chang SM, Dirven L, Lim M, Monje M, Reifenberger G. Glioma. Nat Rev Dis Primers. 2024 May 9;10(1):33
2. Perry JR et al. Short-Course Radiation plus Temozolomide in Elderly Patients with Glioblastoma. N Engl J Med. 2017 Mar 16;376(11):1027-1037
3. Greenberg MS. Greenberg's Handbook of Neurosurgery, Tenth Edition. Thieme Medical Publishing Group. 2023.

Samuel Adida

Thieme

Intracranial Atherosclerotic Disease

1:4

Adults over the age of >25 will have a stroke in their lifetime

Influential clinical trials:

- WASID: Found that aspirin is more effective than warfarin for preventing recurrent strokes
- SAMMPRIS: Showed that aggressive medical therapy outperformed stenting
- MTIAS: Examined the role of medical management in preventing strokes
- VASCULAR: Assessed the vascular effects of intracranial atherosclerosis on stroke risk
- ISS-RS: Focused on intracranial stenosis as a recurrent stroke risk factor

ETIOLOGY

- Intracranial atherosclerotic disease (ICAD) affects the proximal intracranial arteries, most commonly the M1, basilar, ICA, A1, and P1, and is typically defined as >50% stenosis
- Ischemia may result from artery-to-artery embolism, atheroma encroaching on perforator ostia, thrombosis at the site of atheroma, and chronic hypoperfusion due to luminal narrowing

PRESENTATION

- ICAD may be an incidental finding or identified during imaging workup for TIA or ischemic stroke
- Patients may also present with progressive cognitive decline due to chronic white matter ischemia
- The differential diagnoses of luminal vessel narrowing in the context of neurological symptoms include vasculitis, dissection, fibromuscular dysplasia, and reversible cerebral vasoconstriction syndrome

IMAGING HALLMARKS

- Doppler flow studies and vascular stenosis identified on CTA, MRA, or DSA may be used to characterize ICAD

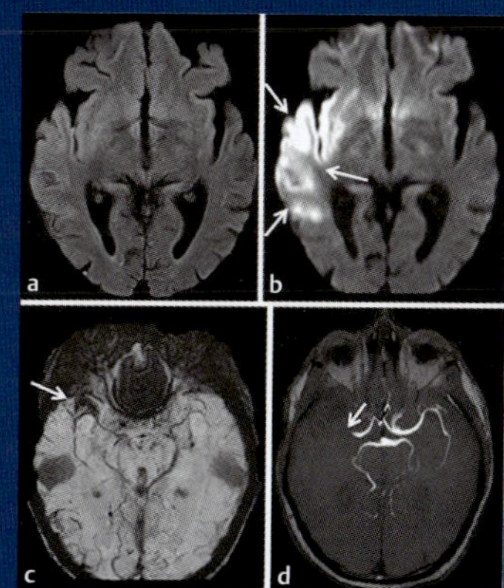

(a) FLAIR sequence in a patient with left hemiparesis. (b) DWI reveals cytotoxic edema in the right MCA territory. (c) SWI and (d) MRA reveal evidence of a proximal thrombus

TREATMENT

- Antithrombotic Therapy
  - WASID showed that warfarin was associated with significantly higher rates of adverse events and provided no benefit over aspirin
- Antiplatelet Agents
  - Aspirin remains the standard therapy. Clopidogrel and cilostazol show potential but lack evidence of superiority. TOSS-II explored aspirin with cilostazol or clopidogrel
- Risk Factor Management
  - WASID suggests LDL <70 mg/dL and systolic BP <140 mmHg should be targeted. There is a lack of evidence for permissive hypertension
- Endovascular Therapies
  - Angioplasty is associated with high restenosis rates (24–50%) and procedural risks. Recurrent stenosis rates after stenting (25–32%) are often asymptomatic. SAMMPRIS found that aggressive medical management is superior to percutaneous transluminal angioplasty and stenting

Further Reading

1. Wang Y, Meng R, Liu G et al. Intracranial atherosclerotic disease. Neurobiol Dis 2019;124:118–132
2. Turan TN, Derdeyn CP, Fiorella D et al. Treatment of atherosclerotic intracranial arterial stenosis. Stroke 2009;40(6):2257–2261.
3. Greenberg MS. Greenberg's Handbook of Neurosurgery. 10th ed. Stuttgart, Germany: Thieme Medical Publishing Group; 2023

Nitin Agarwal
David T. Fernandes Cabral
Samuel Adida

Thieme

Intracerebral Hemorrhage (ICH)-Part I

ICH is the second most common form of stroke (15–30% of strokes) but is the deadliest

OVERVIEW

- Intracerebral hemorrhage (ICH) is a hemorrhage within the brain parenchyma
- Approximately 12–15 cases per 100,000/y
- Diagnosis and management of ICH is a medical emergency
- Risk factors:
    - Age: Incidence increases significantly after age 55and doubles with each decade of life until age >80 y, where the incidence is 25 times that of the previous decade
    - Gender: More common in men
    - Race: In the United States, black > white
    - Previous stroke increases risk 23:1
    - Alcohol consumption
    - Cigarette use
    - Street drugs
    - Liver dysfunction
- Common sites of spontaneous ICH:
    - Lenticulostriates
    - Thalamoperforators
    - Paramedian branches of BA
    - Intraventricular hemorrhage (45%)

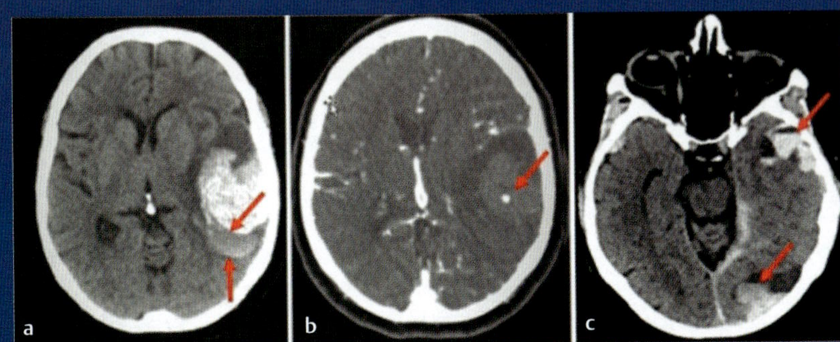

(a) Noncontrast CT scan of the lend sign, showing two differing densities of ICH.
(b) Contrasted CTA showing the spot sign with a hyperdense spot of contrast extravasation.
(c) Fluid–blood level seen in multifocal ICH related to anticoagulant use

Further Reading

1. Sarma A, Ghoshal S, Craven S, Sarwal A. Intracerebral Hemorrhage: a brief evidence-based review of common etiologies, mechanisms of secondary injury, and medical and surgical management. J Neuroanaesth Crit Care 2019;06(02):119–130

Nitin Agarwal
David T. Fernandes Cabral
Samuel Adida

Thieme

Intracerebral Hemorrhage (ICH)-Part II

Hemorrhage expansion occurs in up to 30–40% of cases within the first 24 h and is a major predictor of poor outcomes. Early blood pressure control (target SBP <140 mm Hg) with agents like nicardipine is crucial to minimize expansion

CLINICAL PRESENTATION

General Symptoms
- Headache: Acute, severe, localized, or diffuse, often described as pressure-like or "thunderclap."
- Nausea and vomiting: Owing to increased ICP or brainstem involvement
- Altered mental status
- Motor symptoms, sensory deficits, speech changes
- Cerebellar symptoms: Vertigo, ataxia, dysmetria, and rapid neurological decline with compression of the fourth ventricle

Signs of Increased ICP
- Cushing's triad: Hypertension, bradycardia, and irregular respirations indicating impending herniation
- Papilledema: May be present in chronic cases
- Posturing: Decerebrate or decorticate posturing in brainstem involvement

Imaging in ICH
- Initial imaging: Noncontrast CT (NCCT) is the gold standard
    - Findings: Hyperdense lesion with mass effect, surrounding hypodense edema, and potential midline shift
- CT angiography (CTA):
    - Indications: Suspected underlying vascular abnormalities (e.g., arteriovenous malformations, aneurysms) or spot sign indicating active bleeding
    - Findings: Contrast extravasation suggests ongoing hemorrhage and predicts hematoma expansion
- MRI (with/without contrast):
    - Indications: Subacute or chronic ICH, evaluation for underlying lesions (e.g., tumors, cavernous malformations, amyloid angiopathy)
    - Findings: Blood appears hyperintense or hypointense on different sequences (T1, T2, GRE/SWI for hemosiderin)
- Digital subtraction angiography (DSA):
    - Indications: Young patients, lobar hemorrhages, or unexplained ICH to rule out vascular pathologies
- Differentiating features on imaging: Hematoma, hydrocephalus, herniation

Nitin Agarwal
David T. Fernandes Cabral
Samuel Adida

Thieme

Intracerebral Hemorrhage (ICH)-Part III

CT angiography (CTA) may reveal the "spot sign," a marker of active contrast extravasation. Its presence predicts hematoma expansion and guides aggressive medical or surgical management

MANAGEMENT

Acute Stabilization
- Airway management: Intubate patients with GCS ≤8 or those with compromised airway reflexes
- Hemodynamic optimization: Maintain cerebral perfusion pressure (CPP) while controlling systolic blood pressure (SBP)
  - Target SBP <140 mm Hg, per INTERACT2 and ATACH-II, to minimize hematoma expansion. Avoid rapid BP fluctuations to prevent ischemia
  - Nicardipine: Preferred agent for SBP control due to ease of titration and minimal intracranial pressure (ICP) effects. Initiate at 5 mg/h, titrating up to 15 mg/h as needed
  - Alternative agents: Clevidipine or labetalol, depending on availability and patient-specific factors
- ICP monitoring and management: Place an ICP monitor in patients with large hemorrhages, reduced consciousness, or herniation risk. Treat ICP >20 mm Hg with hyperosmolar therapy (mannitol, hypertonic saline) and elevate the head of the bed to 30 degrees

Hemorrhage Control
- Reversal of coagulopathy:
  - FAST: Hemostatic therapy with rFVIIa reduced growth of the hematoma but did not improve survival or functional outcome after ICH
  - RESTART: Found that resuming antiplatelet therapy after an ICH does not increase the risk of recurrent ICH
- Surgical intervention: Indications include cerebellar hemorrhages >3 cm, brainstem compression, or herniation. Surgical intervention based on radiographic features (MLS, hematoma volume), neurological status, clinical presentation, and when medical ICP alone is not sufficient
- For supratentorial ICH, consider craniotomy or minimally invasive techniques (e.g., stereotactic clot evacuation or endoscopic aspiration):
  - Surgical evacuation done to reduce ICP and/or prevent brainstem herniation
  - STICH and STICH II trials: Both studies evaluated the role of early surgical intervention for patients with spontaneous ICH, with STICH focusing on decompressive surgery and STICH II assessing the benefit of early surgery versus medical management. The results of both trials suggested that early surgery does not significantly improve outcomes compared to medical management, leading to a shift toward conservative treatment in most cases

Prevention of Secondary Injury
- ICP and CPP optimization: Continue hyperosmolar therapy and consider CSF drainage via ventriculostomy for hydrocephalus
- Seizure prophylaxis
- Temperature control to maintain normothermia to prevent increased metabolic demand
- Postacute care
- Neurocritical monitoring: Conduct frequent neurological examinations to detect edema progression, hydrocephalus, or secondary complications
- DVT prophylaxis: Begin intermittent pneumatic compression devices immediately. Initiate low-dose heparin or enoxaparin 24–48 h after ICH stabilization

Nitin Agarwal
David T. Fernandes Cabral
Samuel Adida

Thieme

Intraventricular Lesions

(Lateral and Third Ventricle)

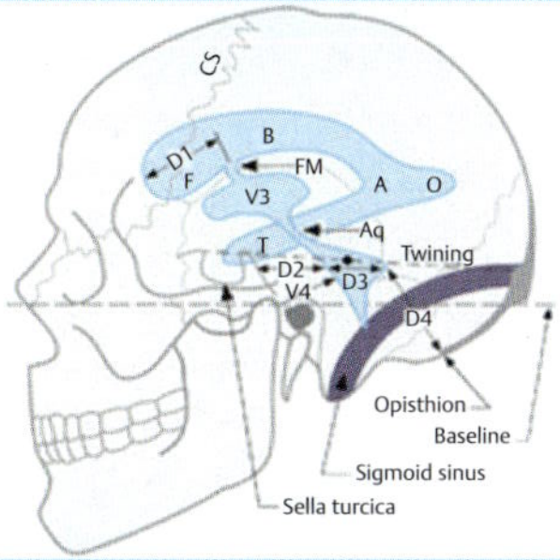

Intraventricular lesions represent 10% of CNS neoplasms

- **In adults, meningiomas are one of the most common tumors in the lateral ventricle**
- **In children, choroid plexus papillomas are one of the most common tumors in the lateral ventricle**

DIAGNOSIS

- Differentiating a tumor located within the ventricle from an intraparenchymal tumor invaginating into the ventricle is a "cap" of CSF surrounding an intraventricular tumor on CT or MRI
- Tumor location, multiplicity, and enhancement can be used for identification

THIRD VENTRICLE MASSES

- Anterior third ventricle:
    - Colloid cyst
    - Sellar mass
    - Sarcoidosis
    - Aneurysm
    - Hypothalamic glioma
    - Histiocytosis
    - Meningioma
    - Optic glioma
- Posterior third ventricle:
    - Pinealoma (dysgerminoma)
    - Meningioma
    - Arachnoid cyst
    - Vein of Galen aneurysm

DIFFERENTIAL DIAGNOSIS

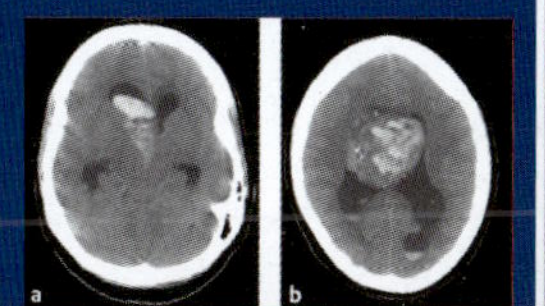

Axial CT scan without contrast of the brain showing an intraventricular mass lesion.

- Astrocytoma (20%)
- Colloid cyst (14%)❧
- Meningioma (12%)
- Ependymoma (10%)
- Craniopharyngioma (7%)
- Medulloblastoma (5%)
- Cystercosis (5%)*
- Choroid plexus papilloma (5%)
- Epidermoid (4%)*❧
- Dermoid (3%)❧
- Choroid plexus carcinoma (3%)
- Subependymoma (3%)
- Ependymal cyst (3%)❧
- Arachnoid cyst (1%)❧
- Arteriovenous malformation (3%)
- Teratoma (1%)
- Central neurocytoma
- Metastases*
- Choroid glioma of the 3rd ventricle

*Multiple Lesions are more suggestive of these diagnosis

❧All lesions enhance except for cysts

SURGICAL APPROACH

Approaches to lateral ventricle:
- Atrium
    - Middle temporal gyrus
    - Lateral temporal parietal
    - Superior parietal occipital
    - Transcallosal
    - Transtemporal horn
    - Occipital lobe incision
- Frontal horn: middle frontal gyrus
- Midventricular body
    - Transcallosal
    - Middle frontal gyrus
- Temporal horn
    - Middle frontal gyrus
    - Transtemporal horn

Approaches to third ventricle:
- Transcortical: Only feasible in presence of hydrocephalus
- Transcallosal
- Subfrontal
- Transsphenoidal
- Subtemporal
- Stereotactic

Further Reading
1. Greenberg MS. Greenberg's Handbook of Neurosurgery. 10th ed. Stuttgart, Germany: Thieme Medical Publishing Group; 2023
2. Nader R, Sabbagh A, Elbabaa S, Al-Jehani H, Gasco J, Gragnaniello C eds. Central Neurocytoma. In Neurosurgery Case Review: Questions and Answers (2nd ed.). Noida: Thieme; 2020

Nitin Agarwal
David T. Fernandes Cabral
Regan Shanahan

Thieme

Ischemic Strokes

Hyperdense MCA sign

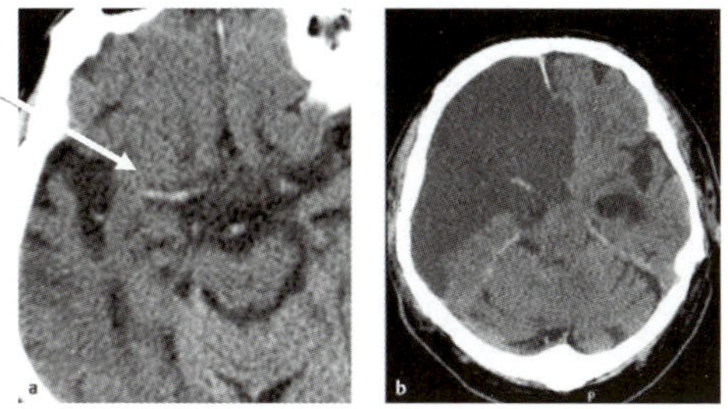

Noncontrast CT of a R MCA stroke at (a) presentation and (b) 2 days post-op

- **Presents with focal neurological deficits based on affected vascular territory:**
  - **Dominant hemisphere (usually L MCA): Hemiparesis, hemianesthesia, aphasia, and R homonymous hemianopia**
  - **Nondominant hemisphere (usually R MCA): Hemispatial neglect, L homonymous hemianopia, anosognosia, and constructional apraxia**
- **Assessment and triage:**
  - **NIHSS and ASPECTS: Evaluate stroke severity and guide management**
  - **Noncontrast CT: Rule out hemorrhage**
  - **CTP and CTA: Assess vessel occlusion, collateral circulation, and ischemic penumbra**
  - **DWI: Detect acute ischemia**

BACKGROUND

- Risk factors:
  - Nonmodifiable: Age and sex; genetic causes (e.g., CADASIL, CARASIL)
  - Modifiable (INTERSTROKE study): HTN (strongest risk), low physical activity, poor diet, obesity, smoking, diabetes, alcohol, and dyslipidemia
- Etiology:
  - Atherosclerosis: Emboli from plaque, especially in the ICA
  - Small vessel disease: HTN causing lacunar strokes
  - Arterial dissection: Intimal tears may cause occlusion or distal embolization
  - Cardiac: Atrial fibrillation, PFO, infective endocarditis, and ventricular wall hypokinesis may predispose to embolism
  - Hypercoagulability: Sickle cell anemia, essential thrombocytosis, and antiphospholipid syndrome
  - Cryptogenic

TREATMENT

Central illustration: Algorithm for triaging patients with acute ischemic stroke with different imaging options

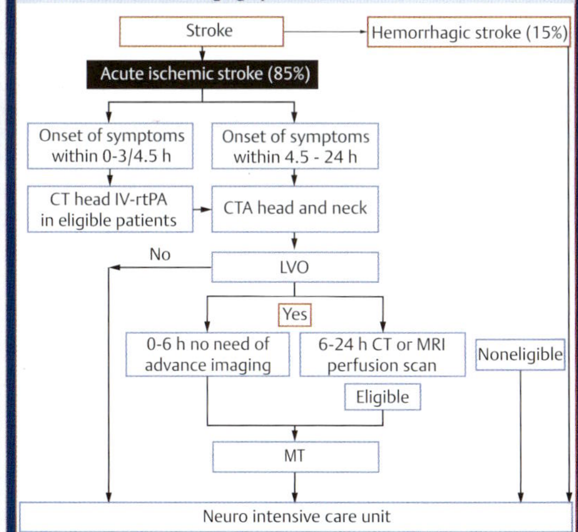

Patel, P. et al. J Am Coll Cardiol. 2020;75(15):1844-56.

- The NIH Stroke Scale (NIHSS) and the Alberta Stroke Program Early CT Score (ASPECTS) assess stroke severity. CT signs include the hyperdense MCA sign and MCA dot signs
- Complications of ischemic stroke include cerebral edema, especially after large infarcts. May require hemicraniectomy to relieve ICP
- Blood pressure management is critical poststroke; avoid hypotension in the acute phase and HTN during recovery
- Antiplatelet therapy (e.g., aspirin, clopidogrel) and statins prevent further ischemic events. In atrial fibrillation, anticoagulation (e.g., warfarin, DOACs) reduces recurrent stroke risk
- Reperfusion therapy with tPA (e.g., alteplase, tenecteplase) is recommended within 3–4.5 h of symptom onset. For large vessel occlusions, endovascular thrombectomy within 6–24 h (DAWN trial) improves outcomes but carries risks like hemorrhagic transformation

Further Readings

1. Campbell BCV, De Silva DA, Macleod MR, et al. Ischaemic stroke. Nat Rev Dis Primers. 2019 Oct 10;5(1):70
2. Greenberg MS. Greenberg's Handbook of Neurosurgery. 10th ed. New York, NY: Thieme Medical Publishing Group; 2023

Nitin Agarwal
David T. Fernandes Cabral
Samuel Adida

Thieme

Jugular Paragangliomas

Up to 40% of jugular paragangliomas arise from heritable genetic mutations, the most common of which involve mutations in the succinate dehydrogenase (SDH) gene

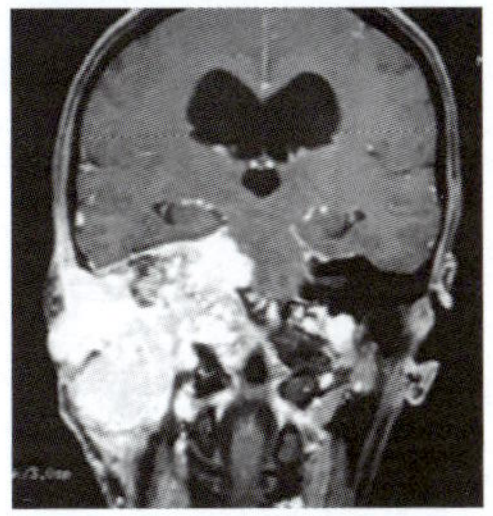

- 50 –60 years
- 5:1 female:male ratio

High catecholamine release can manifest with symptoms such as hypertension and cardiac arrhythmia

PRESENTATION

- Formerly referred to as "glomus jugulare tumors"
- Peak age of incidence: 40–60 years
- 0.6% of all head and neck tumors (~0.07 per 100,000 per year)
- Slow-growing neuroendocrine paraganglioma of the head and neck that arises within the jugular foramen and is localized to the jugular fossa in temporal bone of the skull base
- Neck mass is the most common sign
- Symptoms:
    - Hearing loss and pulsatile tinnitus
    - Lower cranial nerve neuropathy
    - Horner's syndrome
    - Facial palsy
    - Vestibular ataxia
- Potential for malignant transformation
    - 6–19% of glomus vagale tumors
    - 6% of carotid body tumors
    - 2–4% of glomus tympanicum tumors

RADIOGRAPHIC FEATURES

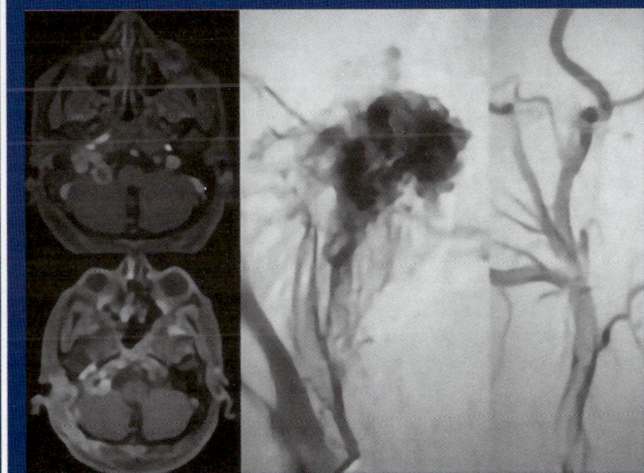

- T1WI: Heterogeneous gadolinium enhancement; typical "salt and pepper" pattern
- T2WI: Tumors are heterogeneous with dark flow voids
- Hypervascular lesion

EVALUATION/TREATMENT

- Evaluation
    - Imaging: DSA, MRI, CT
        - Determine the level of bony invasion
        - Aggressive "moth-eaten" bony destruction
    - Referral to ENT
        - Otoscopic exam
        - Audiological testing
        - Scope to evaluate vocal cord function
    - Referral to endocrinology
    - Plasma and 24-h urine metanephrines
- Observation
    - 65% of the tumors remain stable
    - Serial brain MRI
- Surgical resection
    - Patient managed with alpha-blocker for 2 weeks, beta-blocker 24–48 h pre-op
    - +/– pre-op embolization
- Stereotactic radiosurgery (SRS)
- Subtotal resection + SRS

Further Readings
1. Constanzo F, Nogueira GF, Coelho Neto M, Ramina R. Historical aspects and surgical nuances on the craniocervical approach to the jugular foramen. Arq Bras Neurocir 2022;41(2):174–179
2. Pedro MKF, Leal AG, Ramina R, Meneses MSde. Preoperative endovascular embolization of glomus jugulare tumors: a retrospective case series of 22 embolizations in 20 patients and literature review. Arq Bras Neurocir 2022;41(1):26–34

Nitin Agarwal
David T. Fernandes Cabral
Regan Shanahan

Thieme

Langerhans Cell Histiocytosis (LCH)

Presents with tender lytic bone lesions that involves both the inner and outer skull table and the spine

Diabetes insipidus (DI) can be the first symptom of LCH, and up to 50% of patients with multisystem LCH may develop it

Presents as a multifocal or multisystem disease in children and young adults, with localized disease having a better prognosis

SYNDROMES

- Eosinophilic granuloma
  - Age 5–15 years
  - Single tumors most commonly to the clavicle, pelvis, and spine
- Hand–Schüller–Christian disease
  - Age 5 years
  - Diabetes insipidus, exophthalmos, and skull lesions
- Letterer–Siwe disease
  - Age < 3 years
  - Skin lesions, enlarged liver, spleen and lymph nodes, anemia, and bleeding tendencies

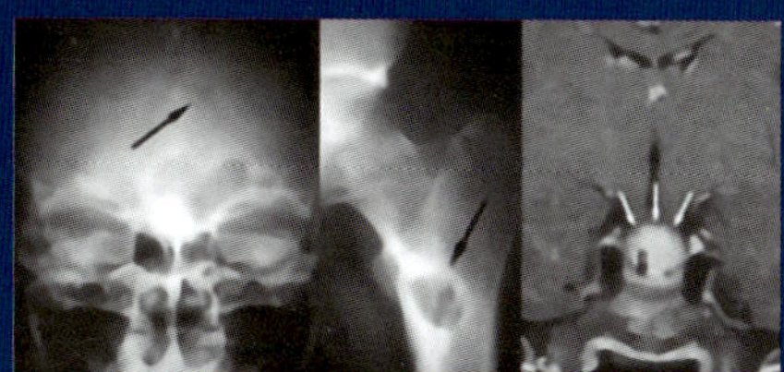

RADIOGRAPHIC FEATURES

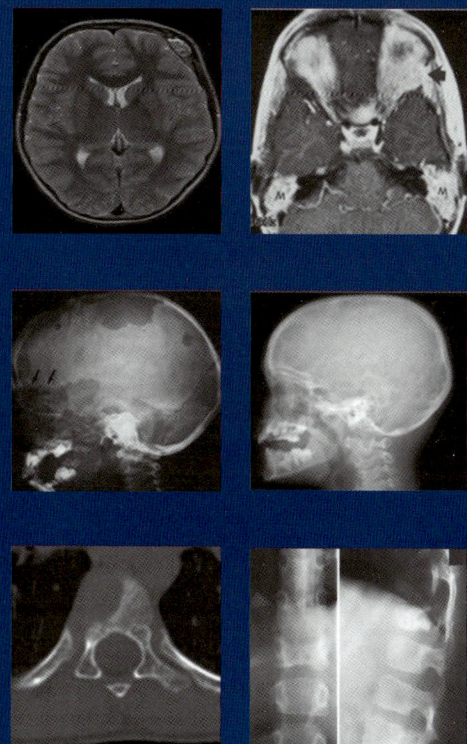

TREATMENT

- "Watchful waiting"—regular monitoring
- Biopsy is required for diagnosis and exclusion of other intracranial lesions
- Combination of chemotherapy, radiation therapy, corticosteroids, and surgery

Langerhans cell histiocytosis

▷ ESSENTIAL TREATMENTS ◁

- **Chemotherapy:** Often used to target and reduce the number of abnormal Langerhans cells; common drugs include vinblastine and prednisone
- **Steroids:** Used to reduce inflammation and suppress the immune system
- **Radiation therapy:** Applied in cases where the disease is localized and not responding to other treatments
- **Surgery:** Sometimes necessary to remove isolated lesions

▷ DESIRABLE TREATMENTS ◁

- **Targeted therapy:** Drugs like vemurafenib target specific genetic mutations (e.g., BRAF V600E mutation) found in some LCH patients
- **Immunotherapy:** Treatments that help boost the body's immune system to fight the disease
- **Bisphosphonates:** Used to treat bone lesions and reduce bone pain
- **Supportive care:** Includes pain management, physical therapy, and psychological support to improve the quality of life

- Resection may be indicated to address lesions to the spine and prevent consequences of kyphosis

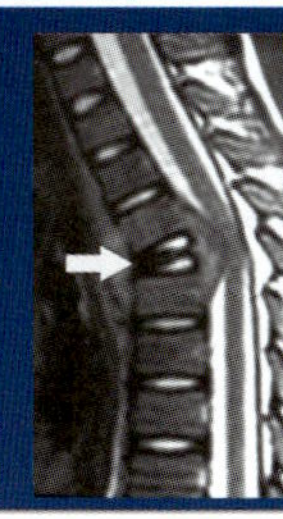

Further Readings

1. Gersey ZC, Zheng I, Bregy A, Agarwal N, Komotar RJ. Intracranial Langerhans cell histiocytosis: a review. Interdiscip Neurosurg 2020;21:100729
2. Huang WD, Yang XH, Wu ZP, et al. Langerhans cell histiocytosis of spine: a comparative study of clinical, imaging features, and diagnosis in children, adolescents, and adults. Spine J 2013;13(9):1108–1117

Nitin Agarwal
David T. Fernandes Cabral
Regan Shanahan

Thieme

Medulloblastomas

Molecular subgroups:
- WNT (MBWNT)
- Sonic Hedgehog (MBSHH)
- Group 3 (MBGrp3)
- Group 4 (MBGrp4)

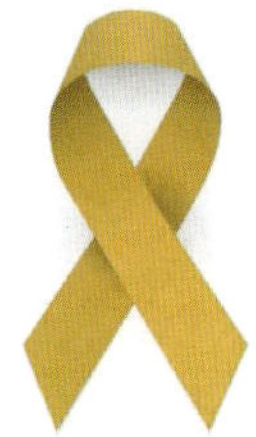

Most common pediatric brain malignancy

WNT is most favorable prognosis: Winning it!
Group 3: The worst

DESCRIPTION

- Tumor type: Embryonal neuroepithelial tumor of the cerebellum (WHO Grade IV)
- Epidemiology: Twenty percent of all pediatric brain tumors, most common malignant pediatric brain tumor; 30–40% of pediatric posterior fossa tumors
- Clinical presentation:
    - Rapid onset of cerebellar signs (e.g., clumsiness, gait disturbances), obstructive hydrocephalus, morning headaches, nausea/vomiting, double vision, and/or blurry vision
- Tumor location: Cerebellum/fourth ventricle

RADIOGRAPHIC FEATURES

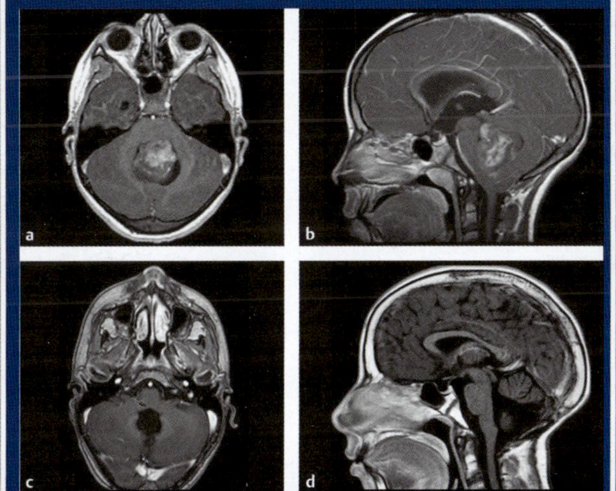

Imaging modalities: CT/MRI
- Solid, midline, contrast enhancing lesion
- DWI restricting on MRI

EVALUATION/TREATMENT

- Differential diagnosis: choroid plexus carcinoma, Ependymoma, Teratoma
- Spinal MRI with gadolinium used to rule out “drop mets”
    - 10–35% experience spinal cord seeding
    - LP is used to rule out seeding ahead of surgery
- First-line surgical debulking
    - Highly radiosensitive and moderately chemosensitive
- In pediatric patients:
    - If >3 chemotherapy and whole axis XRT
    - If <3 chemotherapy until they are three, then XRT.
- 30–40% of children require VP shunts following resection

Further Reading
1. Spetzler RF, Kalani MYS, Lawton MT eds. Surgery of the Brainstem. 1st ed. New York: Thieme; 2019

Nitin Agarwal
David T. Fernandes Cabral
Regan Shanahan

Thieme

Mesial Temporal Lobe Epilepsy

Most common form of drug-resistant epilepsy, often associated with hippocampal sclerosis, focal cortical dysplasia, and epilepsy-associated tumors

Surgical treatment, such as anterior temporal lobectomy or selective amygdalohippocampectomy, is highly effective for drug-resistant cases, achieving seizure freedom in 60–80% of patients

Vagus nerve and deep brain stimulation are alternatives for patients who are not candidates for surgery or experience recurrence after surgery

PRESENTATION

- Mesial temporal lobe epilepsy (MTLE) is the most common focal epilepsy in adults, accounting for 80% of temporal lobe epilepsy cases. Onset typically occurs between ages 10 and 20 years, often following complicated febrile seizures or with a familial history. It can be sporadic or familial, especially without mesial temporal sclerosis. Hippocampal sclerosis is the main cause of drug-resistant MTLE, with focal cortical dysplasia and epilepsy-associated tumors as other causes
- MTLE presents with focal seizures, often starting with auras (e.g., nausea, epigastric sensations, olfactory hallucinations), followed by behavioral arrest and automatisms (e.g., lip-smacking). Secondary generalization to tonic–clonic seizures is rare. Differentiation is needed from absence, insular, and occipital seizures
- MRI shows hippocampal atrophy, temporal horn dilation, and signal changes. Presurgical workup includes video EEG, MEG, PET, ictal SPECT/SISCOM, neuropsychological testing, and invasive studies (e.g., SEEG, subdural grids). Findings include temporal hypometabolism, anterior temporal EEG spikes, and memory dysfunction related to the affected lobe

TREATMENT

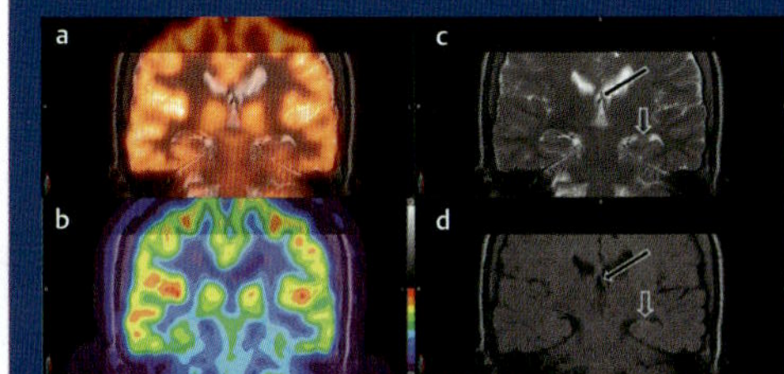

An 11-year-old boy with refractory epilepsy. (a, b) ^{18}F-FDG PET/MRI reveals hypometabolism in the L temporal pole, hippocampal formation, entorhinal cortex, and amygdala. (c, d) T2/FLAIR shows decreased volume and abnormal morphology of the L hippocampus (*open arrow*), with reduced fornix caliber (*black arrow*) and a smaller mamillary body

- First-line treatment: Antiepileptics (carbamazepine, oxcarbazepine, levetiracetam, and lamotrigine, topiramate)
- Surgical options: Anterior temporal lobectomy and selective amygdalohippocampectomy are typically used for medically intractable epilepsy. Seizure freedom is achieved in 60–80% of patients. Postoperative outcomes are classified by the Engel system, ranging from class I (seizure free) to class IV (no significant reduction)
- Minimally invasive procedures: SRS, LITT, and MRI-guided focused ultrasound offer alternatives to traditional surgery, with outcomes comparable to resective procedures
- Neurostimulation: Vagus nerve stimulation and deep brain stimulation are used for patients who are not surgical candidates or experience seizure recurrence, particularly in bitemporal epilepsy or eloquent brain regions

Further Readings

1. Nayak CS, Bandyopadhyay S. Mesial Temporal Lobe Epilepsy. Treasure Island, FL: StatPearls Publishing; 2024
2. Greenberg MS. Greenberg's Handbook of Neurosurgery. 10th ed. New York, NY: Thieme Medical Publishing Group; 2023

Nitin Agarwal
David T. Fernandes Cabral
Samuel Adida

Thieme

Metastatic Brain Tumors-Part I

- In adults, lung cancer, renal cell carcinoma, breast cancer, melanoma, and GI adenocarcinomas collectively account for >80% of brain metastases
- 10% of patients diagnosed with one of these five will develop brain metastases
- 20% of lung cancers result in brain metastases

Sources of cerebral mets in adults (autopsy data)

Primary	%
Lung Ca	44
Breast	10
Kidney (renal cell)[a]	7
GI (colorectal)	6
melanoma[b]	3
Undetermined	10

[a]an uncommon tumor that metastasizes frequently to brain (in 20–25% of cases)
[b]16% in older series "for details, see reference *"
Data from *Greenberg MS. Greenberg's handbook of neurosurgery. 10th ed. New york, NY: Thieme medical publishing group; 2023.

OVERVIEW

- Metastatic brain tumors are the most common intracranial neoplasms in adults, arising from the hematogenous spread of malignant cells from a primary tumor
- The incidence of brain metastases has been rising in recent years due to improvements in cancer survival and detection, as patients with systemic malignancies are living longer
- Intracranial metastases may either be parenchymal (75%) or may involve the leptomeninges in carcinomatous meningitis
- 80% of solitary metastases are ocated in the cerebral hemispheres
- The highest incidence of parenchymal metastasis is posterior to the sylvian fissure near the junction of temporal, parietal, and occipital lobes (embolic spread to terminal MCA branches)
- The cerebellum is a common site of intracranial metastasis, and is the location of 16% of cases of solitary brain metastases (spread via the spinal epidural venous plexus [Batson's plexus] and the vertebral veins)

First-Line Management

- The priority of newly diagnosed brain metastases is the treatment of intracranial edema with dexamethasone and seizure prophylaxis as needed
- Younger patients (<65 years) with high functional status (KPS ≥70), controlled systemic disease, and no extracranial metastases are considered the most suitable candidates for surgery

PRIMARY CANCER

- In adults, lung cancer and breast cancer together account for >50% of metastases
- In children, neuroblastoma, rhabdomyosarcoma, and Wilm's tumor are the most common sources of cerebral metastases

Workup

- Neuroimaging:

MRI: gold standard; features include ring-enhancing lesions, peritumoral edema, and mass effect

  - Multiple lesions and the gray–white junction are typical findings
  - Melanoma, RCC, choriocarcinoma, and lung cancer metastases may present as hemorrhagic lesions
  - Leptomeningeal metastases require contrast-enhanced MRI and CSF analysis for definitive diagnosis

CT scan (noncontrast): May detect hemorrhagic lesions or gross structural abnormalities (e.g., hydrocephalus, midline shift)

- Additional workup:
  - Chest/abdomen/pelvis CT or PET-CT to identify primary malignancy
  - Brain biopsy in cases of unclear primary malignancy or atypical imaging features
  - CSF cytology for suspected leptomeningeal metastasis or high-grade tumors

Further Reading

1. Greenberg MS. Greenberg's Handbook of Neurosurgery. 10th ed. New York, NY: Thieme Medical Publishing Group; 2023

Nitin Agarwal
David T. Fernandes Cabral
Regan Shanahan

Thieme

Metastatic Brain Tumors-Part II

Emergent intervention is required for hemorrhagic metastasis, hydrocephalus, or impending herniation

MANAGEMENT

Surgery

Indications

- Solitary or limited number of lesions that are surgically accessible
- Mass effect causing neurological compromise (e.g., herniation, hydrocephalus)
    - Life-threatening elevated ICP is an indication
- Histopathological diagnosis needed to confirm the primary tumor
- Goal: Maximal safe resection to alleviate symptoms and confirm the tumor's pathology
- Palliative resection may also be an indication
- Techniques include awake craniotomy, neuronavigation, and fluorescence-guided surgery

Radiation Therapy

- Stereotactic radiosurgery (SRS) is the treatment of choice for small, well-defined lesions, typically <3 cm in size or <4 lesions
- Techniques include Gamma Knife, CyberKnife, or LINAC-based systems
- SRS avoids the cognitive decline associated with whole-brain radiation therapy (WBRT)
- WBRT is considered for patients with multiple lesions or leptomeningeal disease
- Side effects: Cognitive decline, especially in patients receiving high-dose WBRT
- May be used palliatively in patients with poor performance status

Systemic Therapy

- Targeted therapy: Agents tailored to the genetic profile of the primary tumor (e.g., EGFR inhibitors, HER2 inhibitors)
- Immunotherapy (e.g., PD-1/PD-L1 inhibitors): Effective in melanoma, non-small-cell lung cancer, and renal cell carcinoma
- Chemotherapy: Limited role due to poor blood–brain barrier (BBB) penetration but may be considered in cases of systemic progression

Supportive Care

- Dexamethasone to reduce vasogenic edema and improve symptoms of mass effect
- Seizure prophylaxis (e.g., levetiracetam, phenytoin)
- Comfort care may be required for patients with advanced disease and poor prognosis

Nitin Agarwal
David T. Fernandes Cabral
Regan Shanahan

Thieme

Moyamoya Disease (MMD)

The most common mutation in moyamoya disease is the RNF213 R4810K mutation, which is found in 90.1% of Japanese patients

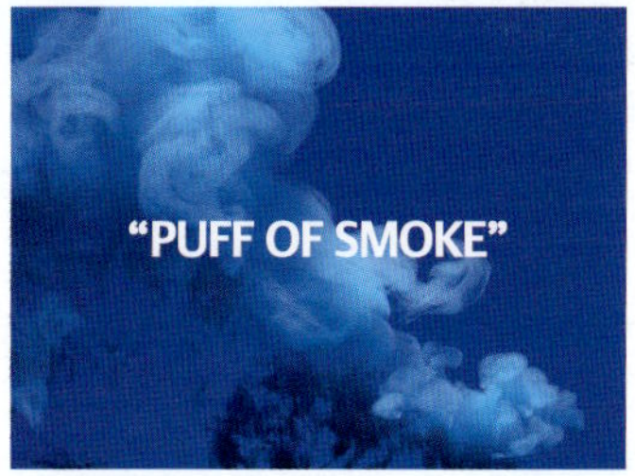

- **Incidence in Japan is higher than in North America**
- **Two peaks:**
  - **Juvenile: <10 years**
  - **Adult: Third and fourth decade**

DESCRIPTION

- Idiopathic, non-inflammatory, non-atherosclerotic progressive vaso-occlusive disease
- Arterial narrowing due to thickened intima
- Progressive spontaneous occlusion of one/both of ICAs
- Intracranial ICA stenosis with concomitant hypertrophic LSA vessels
- Secondary formation of anatomic collateral capillary network at base of brain
- Increased risk of aneurysm
  - Circle of Willis
  - Peripheral cerebral
  - Within moyamoya vessels
- Presentation:
  - Juvenile: Ischemic stroke/TIA
  - Adult: Hemorrhagic (intraventricular hemorrhage due to hypertrophy of anterior choroidal arteries)
- Prognosis of untreated disease is poor, with 73% rate of major deficit or death within 2 years of diagnosis in children, and similarly poor outlook in adults.

RADIOGRAPHIC FEATURES

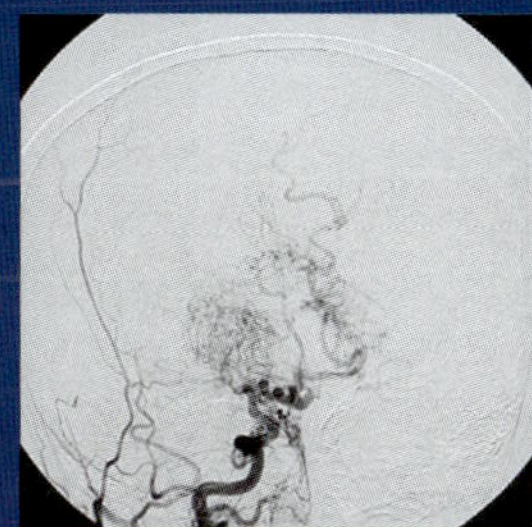

- Carotid angiogram demonstrating moyamoya disease with formation of moyamoya vessels after occlusion of the anterior and middle cerebral arteries
- Imaging characteristics:
  - "IVY sign": Pial collaterals from less affected vessels (especially PCA): forming high serpentine sulcal FLAIR signal intensity and high signal on T1 postcontrast-enhanced MRI
  - "Brush sign": Multiple foci of microbleeds and prominent deep medullary veins on susceptibility sequences

EVALUATION/TREATMENT

- Angiography
- EEG: May show high voltage slow waves in pediatric cases
- CT, MRI, and MRA
- Surgical treatment: Revascularization
  - Direct revascularization
    - Extracranial-intracranial bypass (STA-MCA) bypass
  - Indirect revascularization (pediatric)
    - Encephalomyosynangiosis
    - Encephaloduroarteriosynangiosis
- Perioperative precautions:
  - Avoid hyperventilation, keep $PaCO_2$ 40–50 mm Hg to avoid ischemic infarction
  - Avoid hypotension: Maintain BP at normotensive levels
  - Avoid alpha-adrenergic agents because of vasoconstrictive effects
  - Cerebral protection: Mild hypothermia (32–34° C) and barbiturates can be used
  - Papaverine can help prevent vascular spasm
  - Do not use mannitol
  - Aspirin started on post-op day 1

Further Reading

1. Shaya MR, Gragnaniello C, Nader R eds. Neurosurgery Rounds: Questions and Answers. 2nd ed. New York: Thieme; 2017
2. Mertens R, Graupera M, Gerhardt H et al. The genetic basis of Moyamoya disease. Transl Stroke Res 2021;13(1):25–45

Nitin Agarwal
David T. Fernandes Cabral
Samuel Adida

Thieme

Neurofibromatosis Type 1 (NF1)

Optic pathway glioma (OPG) is the most common brain tumor affecting NF1 patients, predominantly diagnosed in childhood

Genetics:
- **Autosomal dominant**
- **100% penetrance**
- **NFT-1 gene: 17q11.2**
- **Incidence: 1/3,000**

Malignant peripheral nerve sheath tumors (MPNST) most commonly affect the arms and legs

OVERVIEW

- Also known as von Recklinghausen's disease
- Neurofibromatosis type 1 (NF1) is complex multisystem neurocutaneous disorder caused by the mutation of the neurofibromin 1 gene
- Represents 90% of cases of NF
- Diagnosis defined by two or more of the following:
    - >6 café au lait spots
    - >2 neurofibromas
    - Freckling (hyperpigmentation)
    - Optic glioma
    - >2 Lisch nodules
    - Osseus abnormality
    - First-degree relative
- NF-1 causes neoplasms to arise along the nervous system that can grow anywhere on the body
- Overall life expectancy is approximately half that of non-affected individuals
- Tumors or cardiovascular complications are the most common causes of mortality

CNS CONDITIONS

Types of CNS lesions associated with NF1:
- Malignant peripheral nerve sheath tumor (MPNST)
- Glioma:
    - Pilocytic astrocytoma
    - Optic pathway glioma: most common in children < 6 years
    - Diffuse brainstem glioma
    - Spinal astrocytoma and spinal pilocytic astrocytoma
    - Ganglioglioma
- Spinal manifestations:
    - Kyphoscoliosis
    - Posterior vertebral scalloping
    - Hypoplastic posterior elements
    - Enlarged neural foramina

Other malignancies: Gastrointestinal stromal tumor (GIST), pheochromocytoma, myelodysplastic syndrome, osteosarcoma, rhabdomyosarcoma, and leukemia

MANAGEMENT

- Combination of supportive and surgical therapies are employed depending on the specific tumors and anomalies present
    - Optic gliomas:
        - Non-progressive: Followed ophthalmologically and with serial imaging
        - Surgical intervention does not alter visual impairment
    - Other neural tumors:
        - Surgical resection
        - Chemotherapy, radiation
        - Biopsy and internal decompression for malignant degeneration
- Long term tumor surveillance is essential for NF1 patients

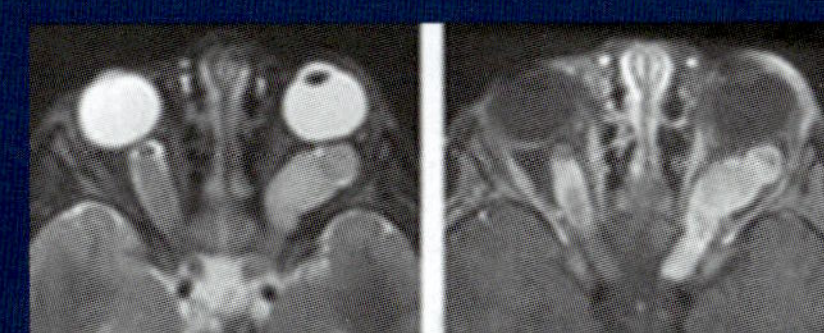

Further Reading
1. Meyers SP ed. Differential Diagnosis in Neuroimaging: Spine. Noida: Thieme Medical Publishers; 2016
2. Mattle H, Mumenthaler M, Taub E eds. Fundamentals of Neurology: An Illustrated Guide. 2nd ed. Thieme Medical Publishers; 2016

Nitin Agarwal
David T. Fernandes Cabral
Samuel Adida

Thieme

Neurofibromatosis Type 2 (NF2)

Approximately, 1 in 50,000 are affected
NF2 is considered an adult-onset disease, the average age of onset is 18–24 years

Genetics

- **Autosomal dominant**
- **50% de novo**
- **NFT-2 gene: 22q12.2**
- **Merlin**

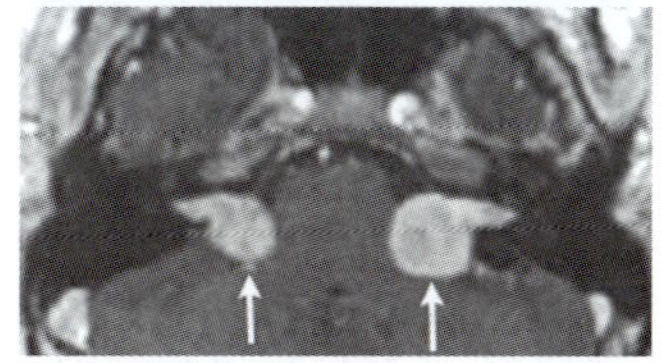

Bilateral CN VIII masses are diagnostic

DIAGNOSTIC CRITERIA

- Neurofibromatosis type 2 (NF2) is a rare autosomal dominant neurocutaneous disorder manifesting as a development of multiple CNS tumors:
    - Intracranial schwannomas (mainly vestibular, sometimes spinal)
    - Intracranial and spinal meningiomas
    - Intraspinal-intramedullary ependymomas
- Unlike neurofibromatosis type 1 (NF1), NF2 is not associated with neurofibromas
- By age of 30 years, almost all affected patients will have bilateral vestibular schwannomas
    - The differential diagnosis for bilateral internal acoustic meatus lesion is sarcoidosis
    - The inferior vestibular nerve is most affected
    - Most patients will become deaf
- Intraspinal tumors are commonly meningioma and ependymoma

OTHER CLINICAL FEATURES

- Seizures or focal deficits
- Skin nodules, dermal neurofibromas, café au lait spots
- Multiple intradural spinal tumors (meningioma, ependymoma, schwannomas down the spine)
- Antigenic nerve growth factor is increased

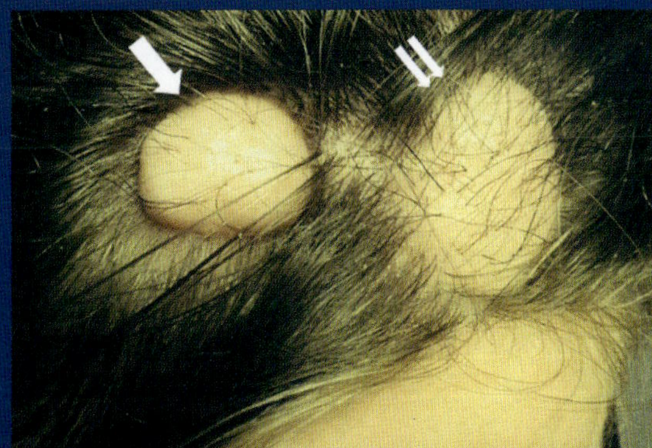

MANAGEMENT

Diagnostic criteria for NF2*
• bilateral vestibular schwannomas (VS) on imaging (MRI or CT)
• OR a first degree relative (parent, sibling, or offspring) with NF2 AND 1. unilateral VS 2. OR any TWO of the following: meningioma, schwannoma (including spinal root), glioma (includes astrocytoma, ependymoma), posterior subcapsular lens opacity, or cortical wedge cataract
• OR unilateral VS AND any TWO of the following: meningioma, schwannoma (including spinal root), glioma (includes astrocytoma, ependymoma), posterior subcapsular lens opacity, or cortical wedge cataract
• OR multiple meningiomas AND ONE of the following 1. unilateral VS 2. OR any TWO of the following: meningioma, schwannoma (including spinal root), glioma (includes astrocytoma, ependymoma), posterior subcapsular lens opacity, or cortical wedge cataract
NB: those with suspicious findings should have molecular gene testing (for details, see reference*)

Data from *Evans DG, Pagon RA, Adam MP, et al. Neurofibromatosis 2. Seattle, WA 1998.

- Bilateral acoustic neuromas
    - Hearing preservation is correlated with smaller tumor
    - Stereotactic radiosurgery therapy may be an option
    - If surgery is indicated:
        - Remove smaller tumor first
        - If hearing is preserved, remove second tumor
        - If hearing is impaired, follow second tumor to prevent total deafness
- MRI of cervical spine is needed to rule out intraspinal tumors that may cause cord injuries

Further Reading
1. Meyers SP ed. Differential Diagnosis in Neuroimaging: Spine. Noida: Thieme Medical Publishers; 2016
2. Carlson ML, Link MJ, Driscoll, CLW et al. eds. Comprehensive Management of Vestibular Schwannoma. Noida: Thieme Medical Publishers; 2019

Nitin Agarwal
David T. Fernandes Cabral
Samuel Adida

Thieme

Occipital Neuralgia

Most common impingement point is the medial branch of the dorsal ramus of C2 or lesser branch of C3

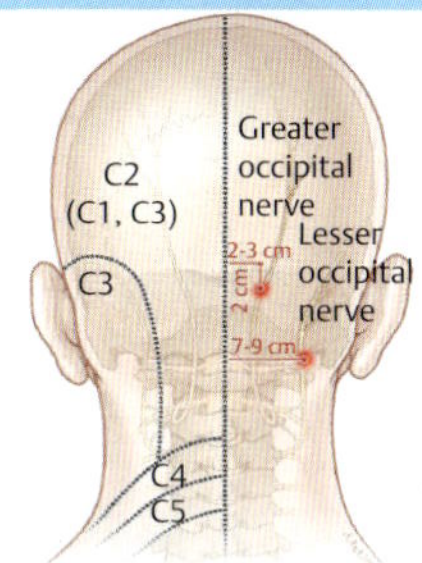

Characterized by severe unilateral pain radiating from the occipital triangle up into the posterior scalp

PRESENTATION

- Greater occipital nerve (nerve of Harnold) is a sensory branch of C2
- Entrapment presents as occipital neuralgia
  - Pain in occiput
  - Trigger point at the superior nuchal line
  - Reproducible pain radiating up along back of heads near vertex
- Differential diagnosis
  - Headache (occipital migraine)
  - Myofascial pain
  - Vertebrobasilar disease
  - Cervical spondylosis
  - Pain from Chiari I

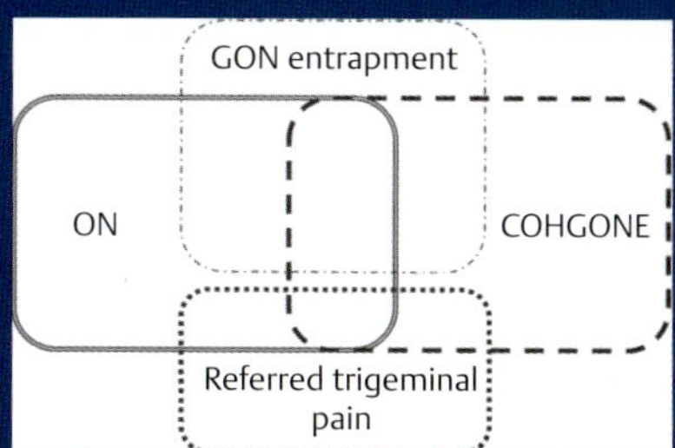

CAUSES OF ENTRAPMENT

- Trauma
- Atlanto-axial subluxation
- Entrapment by hypertrophic C1–2
- Neuromas
- Arthritis

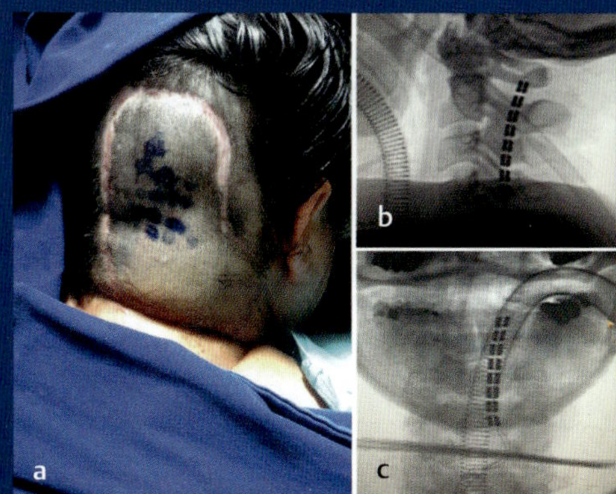

Dorsal cord stimulation for occipital neuralgia

TREATMENT

- Treatment depends on cause and severity
- Non-surgical treatment
  - Greater occipital nerve block
  - Physical therapy
  - TENS unit
  - Oral anti-inflammatory
  - Centrally acting pain medications
  - Botulinum toxin injections
- Surgical treatment
  - Pulsed or thermal radiofrequency ablation
  - Neuromodulation
  - Ultrasound-guided percutaneous cyroablation
  - Surgical decompression
- Dorsal cord stimulator

Further Reading

1. Malheiros JA, Cancado SAV, Oliveira CM de et al. Neurosarcoidosis associated with psychiatric symptoms: case report. Brazil Neurosurg 2017;36(03):200–202
2. Lee C, Son B. V2 trigeminal referred pain from chronic occipital neuralgia caused by entrapment of the greater occipital nerve. Ind J Neurosurg 2019;8(01):76–80
3. Burchiel K ed. Surgical Management of Pain. 2nd ed. New York, NY: Thieme; 2015. https://doi.org/10.1055/b-002-102571

Nitin Agarwal
David T. Fernandes Cabral
Samuel Adida

Thieme

Olfactory Groove Meningioma (OGM)

Genetic risk
- Neurofibromatosis type 2
- Schwannomatosis
- Gorlin syndrome
- Female > Male

Commonly associated Foster Kennedy syndrome (FKS) triad
- Unilateral vision loss
- Optic atrophy
- Swelling in the optic disc of the other eye

Preoperative embolization is deferred due to high risk of blindness from ethmoidal feeder arteries

PRESENTATION

- Tumor type: Benign extra-axial meningeal tumor
- Epidemiology: OGMs represent 10% of all meningiomas
- Clinical presentation: Headache, anosmia, behavioral changes, visual impairment, symptoms of increased ICP, seizures
- Tumor location: Midline of the anterior fossa at ethmoidal cribriform plate
- Insidious growth that can lead to delayed diagnosis and large growth that can cause neurological deficits and impair quality of life

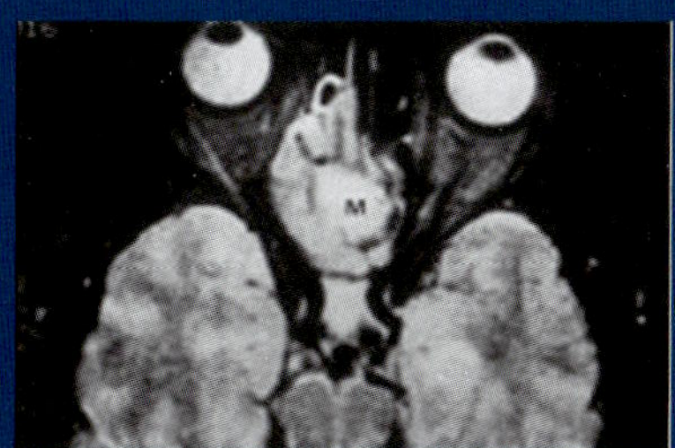

DIAGNOSTIC FEATURES

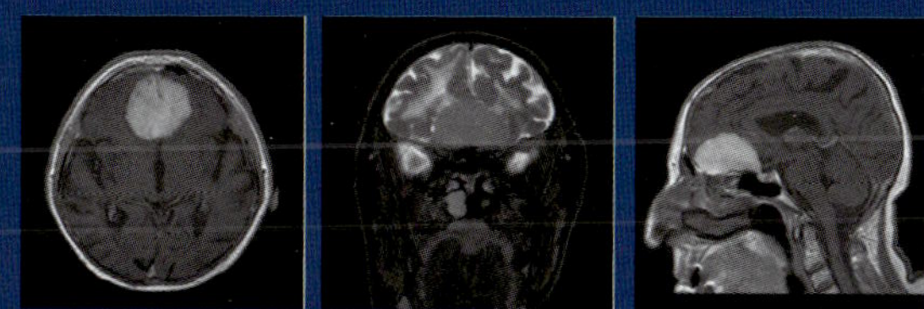

- Imaging Modality: CT/MRI
  - T1: Iso-to hypointense to grey matter
  - T1 C+ (Gd): Intense and homogeneous enhancement
  - T2: Iso-to hyperintense to grey matter
- Histology
  - "Meningothelial" subtype with a proliferation of cells resembling arachnoid cap cells,
  - Whorls with psammoma bodies (calcified deposits) present
  - Low mitotic activity
- Molecular Marker: SMO (Smoothened) gene
- Grading: WHO Grade 1

TREATMENT

- Surgical resection can quickly reduce mass effect, provide early devascularization, and alleviate symptoms
  - Craniotomy
  - Endoscopic Endonasal Approach
- Invasive therapies are associated with post-operative anosmia
- Radiotherapy can be used as an adjuvant treatment
- 5-year recurrence free survival: 88%

Further Reading
1. Yuksel U, Ozdemir A, Kisa U et al. Can routine blood biochemistry parameters be predictive prognostic marker(s) in operated patients with meningioma WHO grade 1? Brazil Neurosurg 2021;40(2):137–145
2. Mastronardi L, Corrivetti F, Bevilacqua P et al. Recurrent olfactory groove meningioma filling the nasal cavity: a case report and technical video. Ind J Neurosurg 2021;10(2):159–161

Nitin Agarwal
David T. Fernandes Cabral
Samuel Adida

Thieme

Oligodendroglioma

Oligodendrogliomas have a bimodal age distribution (peak: 6–12 years, 26–46 years)

Genetically defined by 1p19q co-deletion and IDH mutation (IDH1 or IDH2)

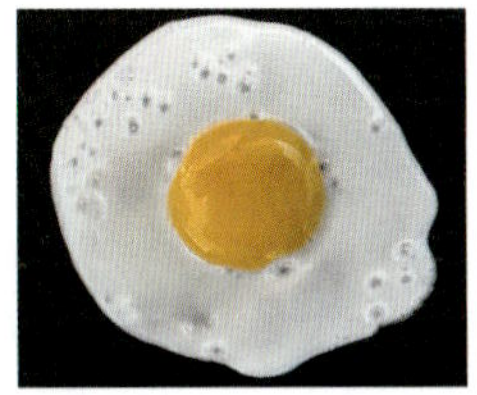

Pathology
- "Fried egg" cytoplasm
- "Chicken wire" vasculature

PRESENTATION

- Nonspecific clinical presentation
- Seizures are presenting symptom in 2/3 patients
- Other symptoms are non-specific for ODG and are more often related to local mass effect
- >50% in frontal lobe
- Calcifications seen in 28–60% of ODGs on plain radiographs, 90% of CTs
- CT: Hypodense to iso-dense
- MRI: Poorly demarcated, hypointense on T1 and hyperintense on T2

GRADING

- Diffusely infiltrating tumor
- WHO grade 2 or 3
- WHO grade 3 characteristics:
  - High cellularity
  - Marked cellular atypia
  - Brisk mitotic activity
  - Pathological microvascular proliferation
  - Necrosis +/− palisading

HISTOLOGY

- Isomorphic with round nuclei and are slightly larger than normal
- Moderate cellularity, arranged in sheets
- 73% have microscopic calcifications
- Permanent pathology shows lucent perinuclear halos with "fried egg" appearance and "chicken wire" vascularity
- Nuclear atypia and occasional mitotic figure is compatible with ODG Grade 2 tumor
- 16% of hemispheric ODGs are cystic
- Usually do not stain with GFAP

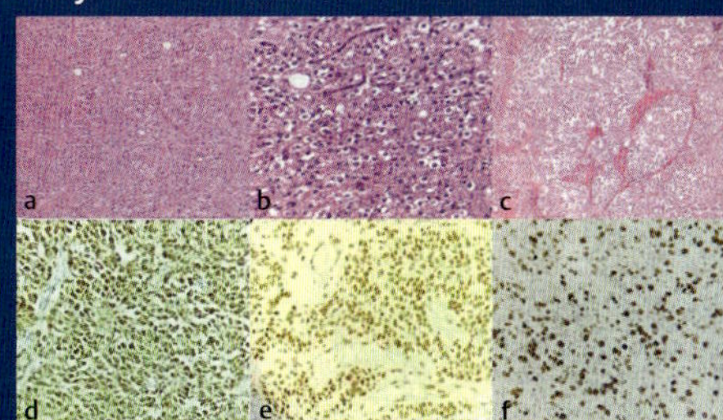

(a,b) Oligodendroglioma showing monomorphic cells with thin plexiform vasculature as well as fried egg appearance of cells and chicken wire blood vessels (H&E stain; x100, x400). (c–f) Anaplastic oligodendroglioma showing increased cellularity and microvascular proliferation, immunoreactivity with IDH1 R132H, ATRX nuclear protein, and a high MIB-1 score (H&E; x100, x400)

RADIOGRAPHIC FEATURES

- Imaging will typically demonstrate a round//oval heterogenous mass with indistinct borders, occasionally cystic, with calcifications
- Symptomatic spinal metastases are very rare

TREATMENT & PROGNOSIS

- Surgical intervention and chemoradiation
- Median survival is 9–10 years
- ODG grade 2 is an independent favorable prognosticator compared to ODG grade 3

Oligodendroglioma, IDH mutant and 1p/19q-codeleted*

▹ Essential ◃

A diffusely infiltrating tumor

And

IDH1 codon 132 or *IDH2* codon 172 missense mutation[a]

And

Combined whole-arm deletions of 1p and 19q

▹ Desirable ◃

- DNA methylation profile of oligodendroglioma, IDH-mutant and 1p/19q-codeleted
- Retained nuclear expression of ATRX
- *TERT* promoter mutation

IDH mutation analysis may not be required when DNA methylome profiling is performed and unequivocally assigns the tumor to the methylation class oligodendroglioma, IDH-mutant and 1p/19q-codeleted.

*Modified with permission from WHO Classification of Tumors Editorial Board, (ed.) World Health Organization classification of tumors of the central nervous system. 5th ed. Bosman F T, Jaffe E S, Lakhani S R, et al. (series eds.): World Health Organization Classification of Tumors series, vol. 6. International Agency for Research on Cancer, Lyon, France, 2021

Further Reading

1. Sharma S, Mathur K, Mittal A et al. Study of surrogate immunohistochemical markers IDH1, ATRX, BRAF V600E, and p53 mutation in astrocytic and oligodendroglial tumors. Ind J Neurosurg 2023;12(02): 137–146

Nitin Agarwal
David T. Fernandes Cabral
Regan Shanahan

Thieme

Optic Nerve Sheath Meningiomas

Benign tumors that often present with progressive vision loss, optic nerve atrophy, and optociliary shunt vessels

Observation is recommended when vision is stable; once vision declines, intervention becomes necessary to prevent further deterioration

RT is generally preferred over surgery due to better preservation of vision and fewer complications

PRESENTATION

- Optic nerve sheath meningiomas (ONSMs) are benign tumors surrounding the optic nerve, making up 1–2% of all meningiomas, 2% of orbital tumors, and 33% of intrinsic optic nerve tumors
- Primarily affects middle-aged women (2:1 female-to-male ratio) and is rare in children (2–4%). NF2 mutations increase incidence (4.1–6.8%), with bilateral cases being rare (5%)
- Present with progressive, painless unilateral vision loss, visual field defects (e.g., central scotomas), dyschromatopsia, proptosis, or diplopia. May also present with optic nerve atrophy and optociliary shunt vessels. The classic triad of vision loss, atrophy, and shunts is rarely seen
- Location is typically orbital but can extend intracranially into the optic canal or sella turcica. Differential diagnoses include orbital schwannoma, optic glioma, orbital lymphoma, inflammatory orbital pseudotumor, and thyroid eye disease

RADIOGRAPHIC FEATURES

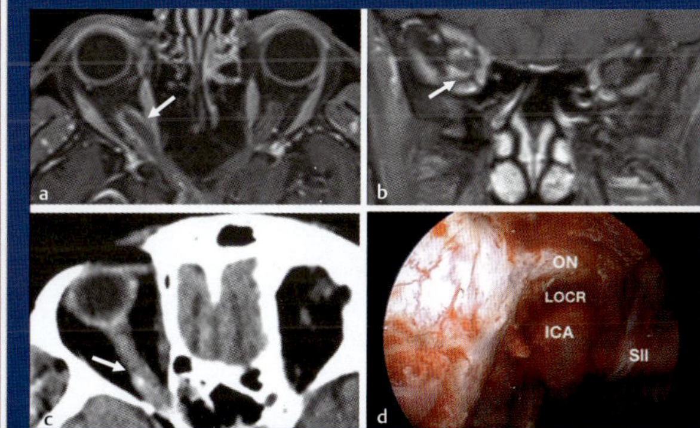

(a) T1 MRI shows circumferential enhancement of the optic nerve, presenting a "tram-track sign." (b) Fat-suppressed MRI demonstrates the characteristic "doughnut sign." (c) CT demonstrates calcifications around the right optic nerve. (d) Resection via an endoscopic endonasal approach, with the internal carotid artery (ICA), lateral opticocarotid recess (LOCR), optic nerve (ON), and sella (SII) visualized

TREATMENT

- Observation leads to progressive vision loss in nearly 90% of patients. Early intervention is associated with better outcomes
- RT has become the preferred treatment, showing superior visual outcomes and lower complication rates than surgery. Various RT modalities including SRS offer targeted treatment with minimal damage to surrounding tissues
- Surgery, while historically the standard, often results in vision loss due to the tumor's blood supply from the optic nerve. Surgery is reserved for cases with no vision, orbital disfigurement, or significant intracranial extension
- Local chemotherapy and systemic therapies have shown limited success

Further Readings

1. Parker RT, Ovens CA, Fraser CL, Samarawickrama C. Optic nerve sheath meningiomas: prevalence, impact, and management strategies. Eye Brain 2018;10:85–99
2. Douglas VP, Douglas KAA, Cestari DM. Optic nerve sheath meningioma. Curr Opin Ophthalmol. 2020;31(6):455–461

Nitin Agarwal
David T. Fernandes Cabral
Samuel Adida

Thieme

Orbital Tumors

Genetics:
- **RB1 gene**
- **NF1 gene**

Clinical presentation:
- **CN III, IV, VI palsy**
- **Vision loss**
- **Proptosis**
- **Diplopia**

- **Most common "intraconal" lesion: cavernous hemangioma**
- **Most common "extraconal" lesion: dermoid cysts (congenital)**

ANATOMY

- Four compartments of the orbit:
  - Ocular
  - Optic nerve sheath
  - Intraconal: Globe, the optic nerve-sheath complex, orbital vessels, and nerves
  - Extraconal: bony orbital walls and fat

IMAGING

- CT remains a strong imaging modality within the orbit
- Less susceptible to motion artifact
- MRI adds information for related extra-orbital structures

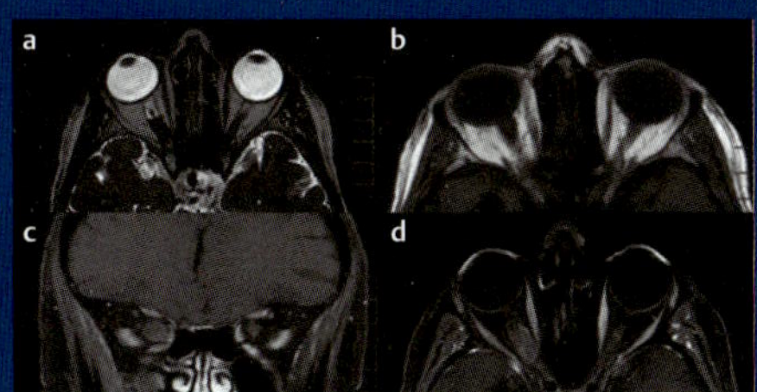

ADULT ORBITAL LESIONS

Differential diagnosis:
- Neoplastic
  - Discrete tumors that may occur adjacent but not envelop optic nerve sheath
  - Melanoma
  - Retinoblastoma
  - Lymphoma
  - Intra-orbital meningioma
- Congenital
  - Coats disease
  - Persistent hyperplastic primary vitreous
  - Dermoid cyst
- Infectious: Toxocara endophthalmitis
- Inflammatory/collagen vascular disease
  - Scleritis
  - Pseudotumor of orbit
  - Sarcoidosis
  - Sjogren's syndrome
- Vascular
  - Enlargement of superior orbital vein
  - Lymphangioma
  - Capillary hemangioma

PEDIATRIC ORBITAL LESION

- Dermoid cyst (37%): Most common pediatric lesion
- Hemangioma (12%): Usually regress without surgery
- Rhabdomyosarcoma (9%): Most common malignant
- Optic nerve glioma (6%)
- Lymphangioma (<7%): Resembles hemangioma

ORBITAL PSEUDOTUMOR

- "Chronic granuloma"
- Idiopathic inflammatory disease confined to the orbit that may mimic a true neoplasm
- Lymphocytic inflammation of the extraocular muscles
- Usually unilateral
- Symptoms: Rapid onset of proptosis, pain, extraocular movement dysfunction
- Usually follows URI
- Steroids are treatment of choice; avoid surgery to prevent further flare

Further Reading

1. Abussuud Z, Ahmed S, Paluzzi A. Surgical approaches to the orbit: a neurosurgical perspective. J Neurol Surg B Skull Base 2020;81(4):385–408
2. Jay A K, Sivanushanthan S, Tsou H, et al. Looking at the eye through an imaging lens: imaging characteristics of orbital lesions for the skull base surgeon. J Neurol Surg B Skull Base 2022;83(S01):1–270

Nitin Agarwal
David T. Fernandes Cabral
Regan Shanahan

Thieme

Pilocytic Astrocytomas

5%

of primary brain tumors

- **Molecular characteristics show BRAF mutations (70–75%) and associations with NF1**
- **Immunohistochemistry is positive for GFAP, S100, and OLIG2, while IDH R132H mutation and p53 protein staining are negative or weak**

- **Gross total resection is the treatment of choice, which is typically curative**
- **RT is reserved for nonresectable or malignant recurrences, while chemotherapy is preferred in younger patients**

PRESENTATION

- Pilocytic astrocytomas are WHO grade 1 astrocytic gliomas, commonly found in:
  - Cerebellum (~60%)
  - Optic pathway/hypothalamic region (~30%)
  - Brainstem (~9%)
- Predominantly affect patients aged ≤20 years (~70%) and are associated with NF1, especially optic pathway and hypothalamic tumors

- Symptom include:
  - Increased ICP: Headache, nausea, vomiting, lethargy, and increased head circumference
  - Other features: Ataxia, horizontal nystagmus, dysmetria, CN VI palsy, and up-gaze restriction

- Imaging shows a circumscribed cystic mass with a brightly enhancing mural nodule:
  - T1 MRI: Solid components iso- to hypointense, cystic components show fluid signals
  - Postcontrast: Vivid enhancement and cyst wall enhancement in ~50% of cases
  - T2 MRI: Hyperintense for both solid and cystic components
  - T2, GRE, SWI*: signal loss in ~20% of cases due to calcifications or hemorrhage

RADIOGRAPHIC FEATURES

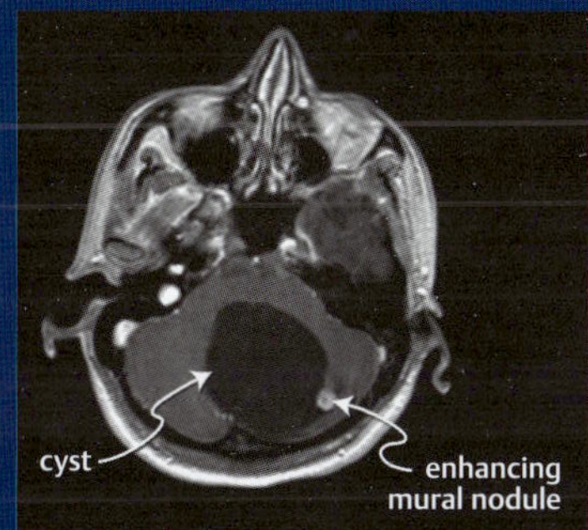

T1 MRI of a posterior fossa pilocytic astrocytoma

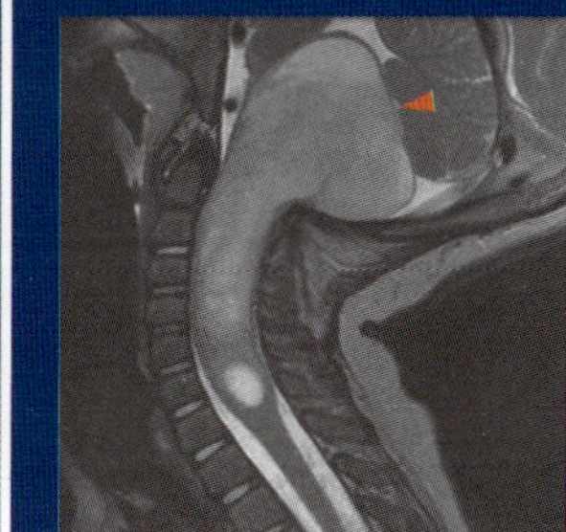

T2 MRI of a 2.5-year-old boy with an expansile, predominantly solid pilocytic astrocytoma. There is a medullary component that results in posterior displacement of the foramen of Magendie indicated with a *red arrow*

OTHER CONSIDERATIONS

- Differential diagnosis includes high-grade astrocytoma with piloid features, hemangioblastoma, and medulloblastoma
- Histopathological hallmarks include a pilocytic appearance with cells having long, thin hair-like processes, Rosenthal fibers (elongated eosinophilic bundles), microvascular proliferation with vessel hyalinization, and low to moderate cellularity

TREATMENT

- The treatment of choice is gross total surgical resection, which is typically curative. In the cases where the tumor consists of a nodule with a true cyst, excision of the nodule alone is sufficient. Following resection, prognosis is excellent, with 5- and 10-year survival rates of 95%
- RT may be considered for nonresectable recurrences or those with malignant histology, although chemotherapy is preferred over RT in younger patients to minimize long-term side effects

Further Readings

1. Knight J, Karsonovich T, De Jesus O. Pilocytic Astrocytoma. Treasure Island, FL: StatPearls Publishing; 2024
2. Greenberg MS. Greenberg's Handbook of Neurosurgery. 10th ed. New York, NY: Thieme Medical Publishing Group; 2023

Nitin Agarwal
David T. Fernandes Cabral
Samuel Adida

Thieme

Pineal Tumors-Part I

Pineal tumors are rare but clinically significant due to their proximity to critical structures. They often present with hydrocephalus, Parinaud's syndrome, and endocrine symptoms

OVERVIEW

- Pineal tumors are neoplasms that arise in or around the pineal gland, a small endocrine structure located in the epithalamus of the diencephalon, situated deep within the brain
- The pineal gland is responsible for producing melatonin, which helps regulate the circadian rhythm
- Tumors of this region are relatively rare but can cause significant neurological symptoms due to their anatomical location and proximity to critical structures, including the cerebral aqueduct, posterior commissure, and tectal plate
- Hydrocephalus is a common complication of pineal tumors and requires urgent management, such as VP shunting or ETV

Etiology
- Genetic mutations: Pineoblastomas may be associated with retinoblastoma (RB1 gene mutations) or Li–Fraumeni syndrome (p53 gene mutations)
- Developmental factors: The pineal gland is a neuroendocrine structure, and disruption in its development could lead to tumor formation, particularly in germ cell tumors
- Environmental factors: Exposure to radiation, particularly cranial irradiation for childhood cancers, has been implicated in increasing the risk of pineal tumors, especially germinomas

Further Reading

1. Pineal tumors. In: Ryan D, ed. Handbook of Neuroscience Nursing: Care of the Adult Neurosurgical Patient. 1st ed. New York, NY: Thieme; 2019

Nitin Agarwal
David T. Fernandes Cabral
Regan Shanahan

Thieme

Pineal Tumors-Part II

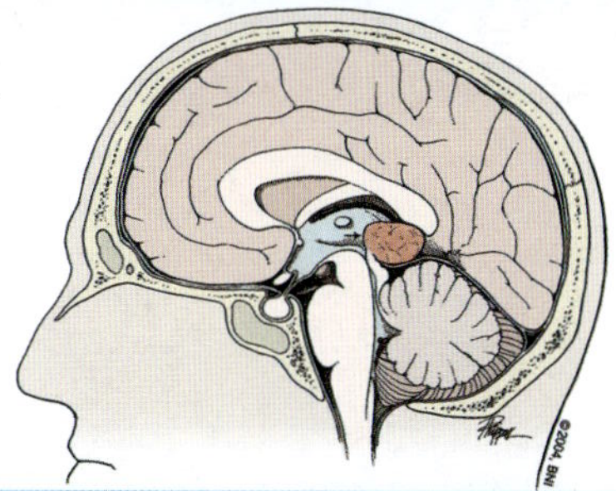

TYPES OF TUMORS

Pineal Parenchymal Tumors (PPTs)
- Pineocytomas: Typically benign, slow-growing tumors. They are often well circumscribed and can be treated with surgical resection
    - 5-year survival: 86–91%
- Pineoblastomas: More aggressive, malignant tumors, often found in children and young adults. They are rare but carry a poor prognosis due to their high rate of metastasis and local invasion
    - 5-year survival: 10–81%

Germ Cell Tumors (Most Common Pineal Tumor)
- These tumors, which can include germinomas, teratomas, and teratocarcinomas, are the most common type of pineal tumor in children and young adults
- Germinomas are typically malignant but highly sensitive to radiation therapy, making them treatable in many cases
- Radiotherapy and chemotherapy are the mainstay of treatment

Metastatic Tumors
- Pineal tumors can also be metastatic lesions, though this is much less common. Breast cancer, lung cancer, and melanoma can spread to the pineal region

Cystic Pineal Lesions
- Many individuals have benign pineal cysts that do not require treatment unless they cause significant mass effect or become symptomatic (typically >2 cm)
- These cysts are often discovered incidentally during imaging for unrelated issues.

Differential Diagnosis
- Colloid cyst
- Metastatic lesions

Nitin Agarwal
David T. Fernandes Cabral
Regan Shanahan

Thieme

Pineal Tumors-Part III

Treatment typically involves surgical resection for benign tumors (pineocytomas), radiation therapy and chemotherapy for malignant tumors (pineoblastomas, germinomas), and hormonal management for endocrine disturbances

DIAGNOSIS & MANAGEMENT

Imaging
- MRI with contrast is the gold standard for diagnosing pineal tumors:
    - T1-weighted images will show hypointense lesions, and T2-weighted images will typically show hyperintense lesions
- MR spectroscopy and PET scans can be used to further characterize the tumor, particularly in identifying malignant germinomas or pineoblastomas

Biopsy and Biomarker
- Surgical biopsy is often necessary to determine the tumor type, especially for germinomas or pineoblastomas, which may require chemotherapy or radiation in addition to surgery
- For germinomas, blood and cerebrospinal fluid (CSF) markers such as alpha-fetoprotein (AFP) and human chorionic gonadotropin (hCG) may be elevated, and their presence can help with diagnosis

Treatment
- Surgical resection is the mainstay of treatment for pineal tumors, especially when the tumor is accessible and nonmalignant (e.g., pineocytomas)
- For pineal cysts that cause mass effect, surgery may also be considered, although these cysts are often benign and require careful monitoring
- In cases of hydrocephalus, a ventriculoperitoneal (VP) shunt may be inserted to relieve pressure before surgery

Radiotherapy
- Radiation therapy is commonly used in the treatment of germinomas (which are highly sensitive to radiation) and pineoblastomas (malignant, aggressive tumors)
    - Stereotactic radiosurgery (e.g., Gamma Knife) may be employed for small tumors or for residual tumor after resection

Chemotherapy
- For germinomas, chemotherapy in combination with radiation is often very effective. Alkylating agents such as cisplatin are commonly used
- Pineoblastomas, due to their malignant nature, may require a more intensive regimen of chemotherapy and radiation

Hormonal Therapy
- If endocrine dysfunction is present, hormonal replacement (e.g., melatonin supplementation) may be necessary to manage symptoms

Nitin Agarwal
David T. Fernandes Cabral
Regan Shanahan

Thieme

Pituitary Tumors/PitNET-Part I

For most pituitary adenomas, transsphenoidal resection is the preferred approach due to its lower risk of complications and better outcomes in preserving pituitary function. Postoperative monitoring for CSF leaks, hormonal deficiencies, and diabetes insipidus is crucial, as these complications can significantly impact recovery

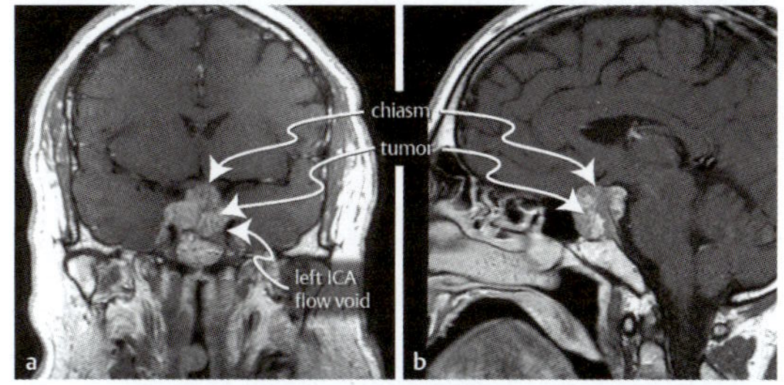

OVERVIEW

- Pituitary tumors, also known as pituitary adenomas, are the most common tumors of the pituitary gland
- They are usually benign but can cause significant clinical manifestations due to their location, hormonal effects, and mass effect on surrounding structures, particularly the optic chiasm

Anatomy
- The pituitary gland is located at the base of the brain within the sella turcica of the sphenoid bone. It has two parts:
    - Anterior pituitary (adenohypophysis): Produces hormones like growth hormone (GH), prolactin, adrenocorticotropic hormone (ACTH), thyroid-stimulating hormone (TSH), luteinizing hormone (LH), and follicle-stimulating hormone (FSH)
    - Posterior pituitary (neurohypophysis): Stores and releases oxytocin and antidiuretic hormone (ADH)

Clinical Presentation
- Mass effect: Headaches, visual disturbances (due to compression of the optic chiasm), and pituitary hormone deficiencies (hypopituitarism)
- Hormonal effects:
    - Prolactinoma: Galactorrhea, amenorrhea in women, erectile dysfunction in men
    - Acromegaly: Enlarged hands/feet, coarse facial features, joint pain, and other systemic effects
    - Cushing's disease: Weight gain, moon face, hypertension, diabetes, and bruising
- Hypopituitarism: Decreased secretion of hormones, leading to fatigue, sexual dysfunction, and deficiencies in thyroid, adrenal, and gonadal hormones

PATHOPHYSIOLOGY

Types of Tumors
Pituitary tumors can be classified based on their size, hormone secretion, and the type of cells they originate from
- Functional (secreting) versus nonfunctional (nonsecreting):
- Functional tumors: These tumors secrete excess hormones, causing endocrine disturbances
- Nonfunctional tumors: These tumors do not secrete hormones but cause symptoms due to mass effect
- Microadenomas versus macroadenomas:
    - Microadenomas: Tumors <1 cm in size
    - Macroadenomas: Tumors > 1 cm in size.
- Common types of functional tumors:
    - Prolactinoma (40%): The most common type, causing excess prolactin secretion
    - Acromegaly/giantism (GH-secreting 30%): Excess GH leading to abnormal growth of bones and soft tissues
    - Cushing's disease (ACTH-secreting, 5–10%): Excess ACTH production leads to hypercortisolism
    - Thyrotropin-secreting tumors (0.5–3%): Rare, leading to hyperthyroidism

Further Reading
1. Greenberg MS. Greenberg's Handbook of Neurosurgery. 10th ed. New York, NY: Thieme Medical Publishing Group; 2023

Nitin Agarwal
David T. Fernandes Cabral
Regan Shanahan

Thieme

Pituitary Tumors/PitNET-Part II

Dopamine agonists (bromocriptine, cabergoline) are highly effective for treating prolactinomas, while somatostatin analogs (octreotide) are the cornerstone for managing acromegaly

DIAGNOSIS & MANAGEMENT

Diagnosis

- History and physical examination: Evaluation of visual field defects (bitemporal hemianopsia), signs of endocrine disorders (e.g., cushingoid features, galactorrhea)
- Hormonal testing:
    - Prolactin levels: Elevated in prolactinomas
    - GH and insulin-like growth factor (IGF-1): Elevated in acromegaly
    - ACTH and cortisol levels: Elevated in Cushing's disease
    - TSH and free T4: Thyroid function tests if thyroid function is suspected to be altered

Imaging: MRI with contrast is the gold standard for identifying pituitary tumors

Management

Medical Management

- Dopamine agonists (e.g., bromocriptine, cabergoline) for prolactinomas
- Somatostatin analogs (e.g., octreotide) for acromegaly
- Steroidogenesis inhibitors (e.g., ketoconazole) for Cushing's disease

Surgical Management

- Endoscopic transsphenoidal surgery: Preferred approach for most pituitary adenomas. It involves access through the sphenoid sinus to remove the tumor
- Craniotomy: Large or multilobar tumors with significant lateral or anterior extension can be approached transcranially

Radiotherapy

- Considered for residual tumors after surgery or in patients who are not candidates for surgery
- Stereotactic radiosurgery (e.g., Gamma Knife) can be used for smaller, inaccessible tumors

Postoperative Care

- Monitor for signs of postoperative complications such as cerebrospinal fluid leaks, diabetes insipidus, or pituitary apoplexy
- Hormonal replacement therapy may be required for hypopituitarism

Complications

- Pituitary apoplexy: Sudden hemorrhage into the pituitary tumor can lead to rapid neurological deterioration and endocrine crisis
- Visual disturbances: Owing to compression of the optic chiasm
- Hypopituitarism: Can occur following surgery or radiation, requiring lifelong hormone replacement
- Recurrent tumors: Pituitary tumors may recur after surgery or radiotherapy, necessitating ongoing monitoring

Nitin Agarwal
David T. Fernandes Cabral
Regan Shanahan

Thieme

Sphenoid Wing Meningioma

EPIDEMIOLOGY
14–20% of intracranial meningiomas

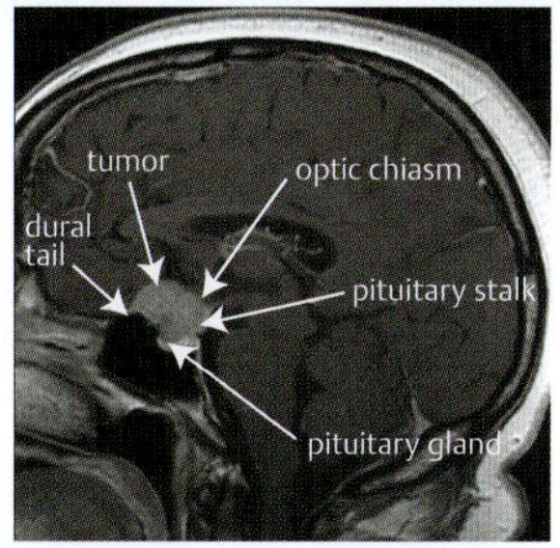

CLINICAL PRESENTATION **Headache, anosmia, behavioral changes, visual impairment, symptoms of increased ICP, seizures**

OVERVIEW

- Behavior and treatment are usually similar to convexity meningioma
- Tumor type: Benign extra-axial meningeal tumor
- Epidemiology: 14–20% of intracranial meningiomas
- Tumor type/location:
  - Globoid tumors (nodular)

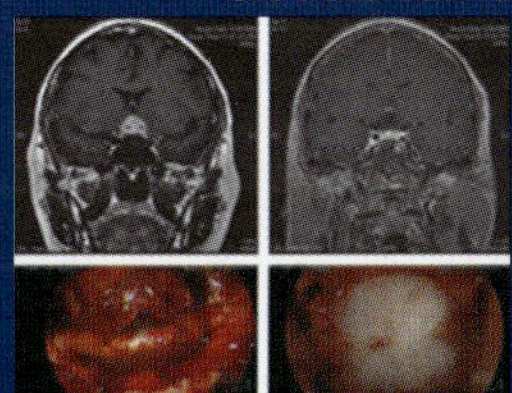

    - Lateral (pterional)
    - Middle (alar)
    - Medial (clinoidal)
    - Tend to encase the ICA and the MCA as well as cranial nerves in and around the SOF
  - Spheno-orbital/hyperostotic (en plaque; flat along sphenoid ridge; rare)
  - Intraosseous (controversial)
- Contrast-enhanced coronal MRI scan preoperatively shows the anterior cerebral arteries (ACA) encased by the tumor as well as invasion in the optic canals. (b) Postoperatively the tumor is completely removed. (c) Intraoperative image shows the postresection bed following opening of the optic canals and removal of intracanalicular tumor from within the sphenoid sinus as well as the ACAs free of tumor.

RADIOGRAPHIC FEATURES

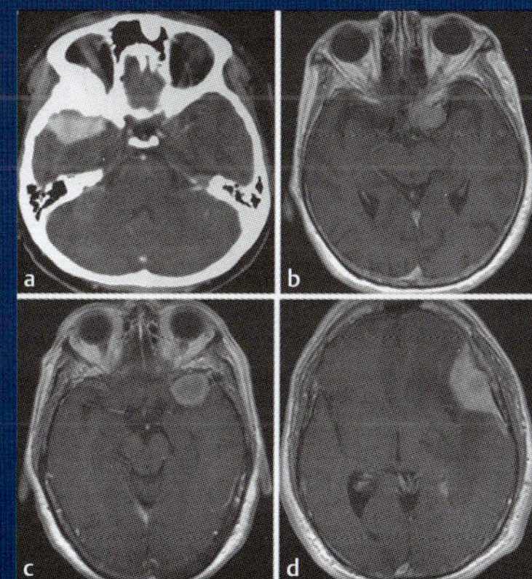

- (a) Sphenoid, (b) clinoid, (c) alar, and (d) pterional

- Imaging modality: CT/MRI with/without contrast
- Imaging hallmarks:
  - T1: Iso- to hypointense to gray matter
  - T1 C+ (Gd): Intense and homogeneous enhancement
  - T2: Iso- to hyperintense to gray matter

CLINICAL MANAGEMENT

- Differential diagnosis:
  - Other skull base tumors like fibrous dysplasia, Paget's disease, osteogenic sarcoma, metastatic cancer, hemangioma, eosinophilic granuloma, epidermoid cyst, and aneurysmal bone cyst
  - Less commonly giant cell tumor, multiple myeloma, or plasmacytoma
- Grading: Typically, WHO grade I/II; biopsy required
- Treatment:
  - Radical surgical excision via the frontotemporal approach (pterional or fronto-orbitozygomatic):
    - Simpson grades
  - Adjuvant radiosurgery for residual tumor
- Prognosis: Generally good with gross total resection:
  - Progression-free survival, 80% at 5 years to 50% at 20 years following complete surgical removal

Further Readings
1. Stamm A, ed. Reconstruction. In: Transnasal Endoscopic Skull Base and Brain Surgery: Surgical Anatomy and Its Applications. 2nd ed. New York, NY: Thieme; 2019
2. Jayashankar N, Narayanan P, eds. Planum sphenoidale and tuberculum sellae meningioma. In: Atlas of 360 Degree Skull Base Surgery. 1st ed. Noida, India: Thieme; 2021

Nitin Agarwal
David T. Fernandes Cabral
Samuel Adida

Thieme

Spinal Chordomas

20%

of all primary spine tumors

- En bloc resection with wide margins is the traditional standard of care, though complete resection is difficult to achieve and often complicated
- Radioresistant tumor and typically treated with high-dose RT in the form of proton beam, carbon ion, and SRS after resection
- Recurrence rates are variable ranging from 35 to 75% after resection

PRESENTATION

- Chordomas are low-grade, slow-growing, and locally invasive tumors arising from remnants of the notochord, a mesodermal structure
- These tumors occur along the midline of the spinal axis, spanning from the clivus to the sacrum. They are most commonly found in the sacrum (50%), followed by the skull base (35%) and mobile spine (15%). Chordoma often affects individuals in the age range of 40–60 years, with a male-to-female ratio of 2:1
- Present with varying symptoms depending on their location:
  - Cervical chordomas may result in neck pain, dysphagia, and lower CN dysfunction
  - Thoracic, lumbar, and sacral chordomas may cause localized pain, pathologic fractures, and radiculopathy or myelopathy

RADIOGRAPHIC FEATURES

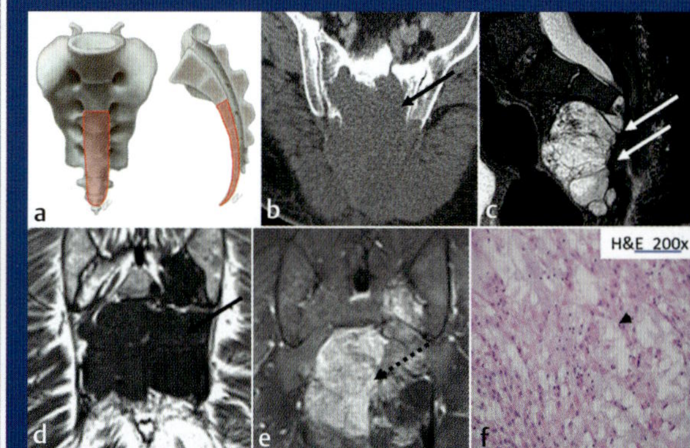

(a) Characteristic chordoma location in the lower sacrum. (b) CT demonstrates the lytic sacral lesion. (c) T2 MRI shows a heterogeneous hyperintense mass and (d) T1 MRI shows a hypointense mass with (e) postcontrast enhancement. (f) Pathology shows large epithelioid cells, including physaliphorous cells with intracytoplasmic vacuoles in a myxoid stroma

TREATMENT

- Treatment for spinal chordomas is surgical resection, ideally en bloc with wide margins
- Complete resection in the spine is often complicated with nerve and vascular sacrifice and may be difficult to achieve due to epidural involvement
- Radioresistant and require treatment with high-dose RT after resection. Proton beam, carbon ion, and SRS therapy may be used as adjuvant treatment instead of conventional RT and may be utilized as primary or definitive treatment
- Chemotherapy is generally not effective
- Given recurrence rates, imaging surveillance is essential to monitor for progression or metastasis. The 5-year survival rate for chordomas is ~50%, but prognosis varies depending on the tumor's location, size, and management

Further Readings

1. Baier MP, Cheong DA, Shi HH, et al. Decision-making in clival mass lesions: risk factors for malignant disease and an illustrative case example. J Neurol Surg Rep 2023;84(4):e156–e162
2. Tenny S, Varacallo MA. Chordoma. Treasure Island, FL: StatPearls Publishing; 2025
3. Greenberg MS. Greenberg's Handbook of Neurosurgery. 10th ed. New York, NY: Thieme Medical Publishing Group; 2023

Nitin Agarwal
David T. Fernandes Cabral
Samuel Adida

Thieme

Subarachnoid Hemorrhage-Part I

Over 85% of spontaneous Subarachnoid Hemorrhages (SAHs) are caused by the rupture of saccular (berry) aneurysms, most commonly located at the arterial branch points of the circle of Willis (e.g., anterior communicating artery, posterior communicating artery, and middle cerebral artery)

OVERVIEW

- Serious and often life-threatening medical condition characterized by bleeding into the subarachnoid space
- *Traumatic SAH*: Often results from blunt head trauma, presenting with localized subarachnoid blood, typically near the site of injury, and may be accompanied by other signs of trauma such as skull fractures or brain contusions
- *Aneurysmal SAH*: Typically presents with a sudden, severe headache (often the "worst headache of my life") and is caused by the rupture of an intracranial aneurysm, with blood usually seen around the circle of Willis on imaging
- Pathophysiology: When an aneurysm ruptures, blood enters the subarachnoid space, leading to an increase in intracranial pressure (ICP) and disruption of normal cerebral blood flow. The presence of blood in this area can cause irritation of the meninges, leading to inflammation, vasospasm (narrowing of blood vessels), and reduced oxygen supply to brain tissues
- Clinical grading scales are used to assess the risk of vasospasm
- CONSCIOUS-2 trial failed to demonstrate a significant effect of clazosentan on vasospasm-related mortality

Fisher Grading for SAH
- Grade 1: No blood or minimal blood in the subarachnoid space. Low risk of vasospasm
- Grade 2: Blood in the subarachnoid space, but no significant amounts in the basal cisterns or ventricles. Moderate risk of vasospasm
- Grade 3: Blood present in the basal cisterns or ventricles, or significant clot formation
- High risk of vasospasm
- Grade 4: Diffuse blood throughout the subarachnoid space with extensive clot formation and/or intraventricular hemorrhage. Very high risk of vasospasm, as well as poorer clinical outcomes

Further Reading

1. Merrill S, Sen A. Diagnostic challenges. In: Bendok B, Batjer H, ed. Hemorrhagic and Ischemic Stroke: Medical, Imaging, Surgical, and Interventional Approaches. 2nd ed. New York, NY: Thieme; 2024

Nitin Agarwal
David T. Fernandes Cabral
Regan Shanahan

Thieme

Subarachnoid Hemorrhage-Part II

A noncontrast CT scan detects SAH in over 90% of cases within 24 h of symptom onset. If the CT is negative but clinical suspicion is high (e.g., thunderclap headache), perform a lumbar puncture to look for xanthochromia or proceed with CT angiography (CTA) to identify aneurysms or vascular abnormalities

CLINICAL FEATURES

The presentation of SAH is typically sudden and dramatic. Key symptoms include the following:

- Severe headache ("thunderclap headache"): Often described as the worst headache of the patient's life
- Neck stiffness: Owing to irritation of the meninges
- Nausea and vomiting: Often accompanying increased ICP
- Photophobia: Sensitivity to light
- Loss of consciousness: Can vary from brief periods of confusion to full coma
- Seizures: May occur in some cases
- Focal neurological deficits: Weakness, speech difficulty, or other signs of brain dysfunction may appear, depending on the affected area.

Hunt and Hess Score for SAH

- Grade 1: Asymptomatic or mild headache; no neurological deficits. Good prognosis
- Grade 2: Moderate headache and nuchal rigidity (neck stiffness); no or mild neurological deficits. Fair prognosis
- Grade 3: Drowsy or confused; mild focal neurological deficits (e.g., hemiparesis). Guarded prognosis

- Grade 4: Stuporous with severe focal neurological deficits, hemiplegia, or other signs of significant brain injury. Poor prognosis
- Grade 5: Comatose, posturing, or severe neurological impairment (e.g., decerebrate rigidity)

Diagnosis

- CT scan with/without contrast
- Lumbar puncture
- MRI
- Cerebral angiography

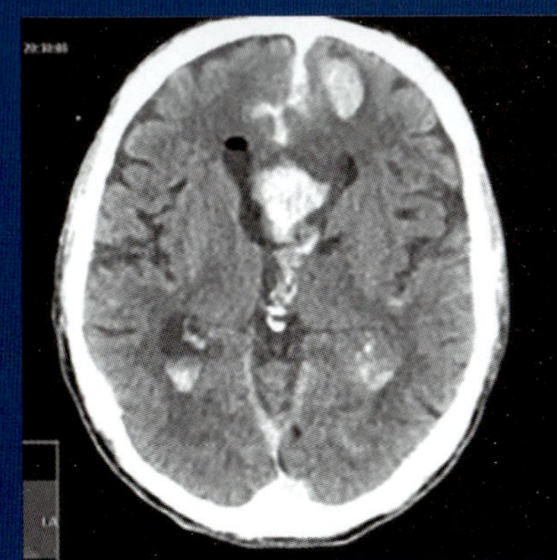

Nitin Agarwal
David T. Fernandes Cabral
Regan Shanahan

Thieme

Subarachnoid Hemorrhage-Part III

Vasospasm typically occurs 4–14 days post-SAH and is a leading cause of secondary neurological deterioration. Prophylactic nimodipine is the standard therapy to reduce DCI risk

MANAGEMENT

Early Aneurysm Treatment (within 1–3 Days)

- Goal: Early securement of the aneurysm (either surgically or endovascularly) to prevent rebleeding
- Early blood pressure (BP) management with nimodipine:
    - AHA/ASA guidelines: Recommend maintaining systolic BP (SBP) <160 mm Hg in aneurysmal SAH (aSAH) before securing the aneurysm to reduce the risk of rebleeding
    - INTERACT2 trial: Suggesting that aggressive BP control reduces hematoma expansion but had no definitive impact on functional outcomes
    - ATACH-II trial: Examined aggressive BP control in acute ICH (target SBP <140 mm Hg) and found no significant improvement in functional outcomes but an increased risk of renal adverse events, suggesting caution in excessively lowering BP in hemorrhagic conditions
    - Ultralow BP study (subgroup analyses in SAH): Some retrospective studies suggest that aggressively lowering SBP <120 mm Hg before aneurysm securing may risk cerebral ischemia
- Treatment options:
    - Surgical clipping: A metal clip is placed on the aneurysm's neck to stop blood flow
    - Endovascular coiling: A catheter is inserted into an artery, and small coils are placed within the aneurysm to clot it off
        - ISAT: For patients with ruptured intracranial aneurysms suitable for either endovascular coiling or neurosurgical clipping, endovascular coiling resulted in better 1-year clinical outcomes, defined as survival without dependency, compared to surgical clipping

Managing Complications (Days to Weeks)

- Rebleeding: The risk of rebleeding is highest in the first few days after the hemorrhage
- Hydrocephalus: SAH can cause a buildup of fluid in the brain, leading to hydrocephalus
- Vasospasm: Narrowing of the blood vessels in the brain can lead to delayed cerebral ischemia (DCI)

Treatment of Complications

- Antifibrinolytics: Medications like tranexamic acid can help reduce the risk of rebleeding
- Nimodipine: A calcium channel blocker that helps prevent vasospasm
- Induced hypertension: Elevating BP can help improve blood flow to the brain
- Volume expansion: Administering fluids to increase blood volume
- Endovascular treatment for vasospasm: Angioplasty or intra-arterial vasodilators can be used to treat vasospasm
- Shunt placement: If hydrocephalus is severe, a shunt may be needed to drain excess fluid

Notable Trials

- STASH: Did not detect any benefit in the use of simvastatin for long- or short-term outcome in patients with aneurysmal SAH

Nitin Agarwal
David T. Fernandes Cabral
Regan Shanahan

Thieme

Subependymal Giant Cell Astrocytomas

Occur in 5–20% of patients with tuberous sclerosis complex

Commonly arises in the foramen of Monro, where it can obstruct CSF flow leading to obstructive hydrocephalus

Management includes surgical resection for symptomatic cases or mTOR inhibitors, such as everolimus, to reduce tumor size in inoperable or asymptomatic cases

PRESENTATION

- Subependymal giant cell astrocytoma (SEGA) is a rare, benign brain tumor typically arising along the lateral ventricle wall, near the foramen of Monro, and occasionally in the third ventricle
- Clinical features: Often asymptomatic early; growth may obstruct CSF flow, causing hydrocephalus, increased ICP, headaches, seizures, ataxia, and visual disturbances
- Diagnosis: Clinical evaluation and MRI show a well-circumscribed, enhancing mass at the foramen of Monro, often with calcifications or cysts. Genetic testing for tuberous sclerosis complex (TSC) mutations may support diagnosis
- Histology: Astrocyte-like, spindle, and giant cells on a fibrillar background, often with calcification. Mitotic activity, pleomorphism, and necrosis have no prognostic significance

RADIOGRAPHIC FEATURES

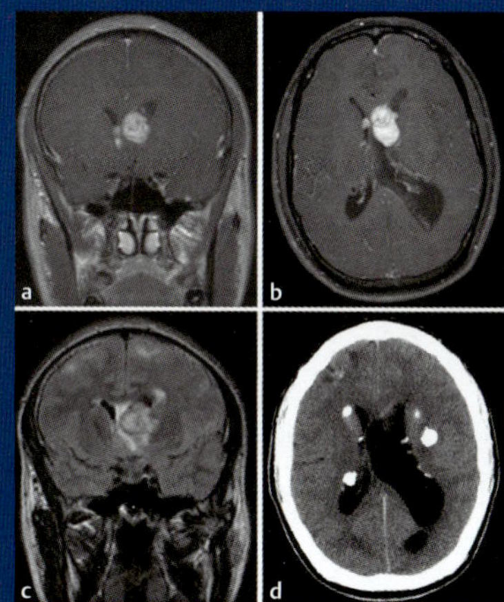

(a, b) T1 MRI, (c) FLAIR MRI, and (d) CT reveal multiple enhancing nodules at the bilateral foramina of Monro. Coarse calcifications suggest subependymal nodules, while subcortical supratentorial lesions show FLAIR hyperintensity and gyral expansion consistent with tubers

TREATMENT

- Surveillance: Essential to monitor progression and prevent hydrocephalus
- Resection:
  - Surgery is preferred for symptomatic tumors; early and complete resection offers the best prognosis
  - Minimally invasive approaches such as endoscopic tumor removal may be considered for tumors <3 cm
- Pharmacotherapy:
  - mTOR inhibitors: Everolimus and sirolimus reduce tumor size, especially in asymptomatic or inoperable cases, and shrink other TSC-related lesions (e.g., kidney angiomyolipomas, cardiac rhabdomyomas)
    - Everolimus has shown significant success in clinical trials, with long-term tumor regression
    - Treatment may need to be maintained indefinitely to prevent regrowth
    - Common side effects include stomatitis, infections, and fatigue, requiring monitoring

Further Readings

1. Pucko E, Sulejczak D, Ostrowski RP. Subependymal giant cell astrocytoma: the molecular landscape and treatment advances. Cancers (Basel) 2024;16(19):3406
2. Gao C, Zabielska B, Jiao F, et al. Subependymal giant cell astrocytomas in tuberous sclerosis complex-current views on their pathogenesis and management. J Clin Med 2023;12(3):956
3. Tahiri Elousrouti L, Lamchahab M, Bougtoub N, et al. Subependymal giant cell astrocytoma (SEGA): a case report and review of the literature. J Med Case Rep 2016;10:35

Nitin Agarwal
David T. Fernandes Cabral
Samuel Adida

Thieme

Transient Ischemic Attack (TIA)-Part I

- **Stroke risk incidence: Approximately 200,000 TIAs occur annually in the United States**
- **10–15% of patients will experience a stroke within 90 days**
- **50% of those strokes occur within the first 48 h, emphasizing the need for immediate risk stratification and treatment**

OVERVIEW

- A transient ischemic attack (TIA) is a temporary episode of neurological dysfunction caused by focal cerebral, spinal, or retinal ischemia, without evidence of acute infarction
- Often termed a "mini-stroke," a TIA serves as an early warning sign of an impending ischemic stroke, with a particularly high risk in the first 48 h to 90 days

1. *Anterior Circulation (Carotid Artery) TIA–MCA/ACA Territory*

Middle cerebral artery (MCA) TIA:
- Contralateral hemiparesis (face, arm > leg)
- Contralateral sensory loss
- Aphasia (if dominant hemisphere involved)
- Contralateral hemianopia (visual field deficit)

Anterior cerebral artery (ACA) TIA:
- Contralateral leg weakness and sensory deficits
- Frontal lobe dysfunction, including abulia (lack of motivation) or personality changes

Retinal ischemia (amaurosis fugax):
- Transient monocular vision loss, described as a "curtain coming down" over the eye
- Typically due to emboli to the central retinal artery

2. *Posterior Circulation (Vertebrobasilar) TIA*
- Diplopia, dysarthria, dysphagia (cranial nerve involvement)
- Ataxia, vertigo, dizziness (cerebellar ischemia)
- Contralateral hemiparesis or sensory loss
- Drop attacks (sudden loss of postural tone without loss of consciousness)
- Crossed signs (ipsilateral cranial nerve deficits with contralateral motor/sensory deficits)
- Homonymous hemianopia or cortical blindness (occipital lobe involvement)

Basilar artery TIA ("Locked-in Syndrome" in severe cases):
- Quadriparesis, dysarthria, and consciousness preserved

Nitin Agarwal
David T. Fernandes Cabral
Regan Shanahan

Thieme

Transient Ischemic Attack (TIA)-Part II

Large vessel stenosis requires surgical consideration: CEA is indicated for symptomatic 50–99% carotid stenosis

PATHOPHYSIOLOGY

A TIA occurs due to a temporary reduction in cerebral blood flow, which does not cause permanent infarction or irreversible neuronal injury. The major etiologies include the following:

- Embolic TIA (most common mechanism):
    - Cardiogenic emboli: Atrial fibrillation, left atrial thrombus, valvular disease (e.g., mitral stenosis, infective endocarditis), patent foramen ovale (PFO)
    - Arterio-arterial emboli: Atherosclerotic plaques from the carotid arteries or vertebrobasilar system may send emboli to distal cerebral arteries
    - Paradoxical embolism: Right-to-left shunting via a PFO allows venous thrombi to bypass pulmonary circulation and enter cerebral circulation
- Thrombotic TIA:
    - In situ thrombosis occurs in small perforating arteries (e.g., lenticulostriate, thalamoperforator arteries), commonly associated with hypertension, diabetes, and smoking
- Hemodynamic TIA (less common):
    - Hypoperfusion due to systemic hypotension (e.g., cardiac arrhythmias, sepsis) or severe proximal stenosis (e.g., carotid occlusion) results in transient ischemia in watershed areas
    - Symptoms may be positional or exertional, and typically resolve with rest

Risk Stratification

- Stroke risk stratification, $ABCD^2$ score predicts early stroke risk:
    - Age ≥60 (1 point)
    - Blood pressure ≥140/90 mm Hg (1 point)
    - Clinical features (unilateral weakness = 2 points, speech disturbance = 1 point)
    - Duration (>60 min = 2 points, 10–59 min = 1 point)
    - Diabetes (1 point)
    - Score ≥4 = high risk (urgent evaluation and intervention needed)

Nitin Agarwal
David T. Fernandes Cabral
Regan Shanahan

Thieme

Transient Ischemic Attack (TIA)-Part III

A positive DWI lesion suggests stroke, not TIA, impacting management

DIAGNOSIS & MANAGEMENT

- Since TIA symptoms resolve spontaneously, prompt evaluation is crucial to prevent a subsequent stroke
- Goals of initial evaluation:
  - Prove vascular origin of symptoms (hypoperfusion and/or acute infarction or large vessel stenosis)
  - Exclude nonischemic etiology
  - Determine the underlying vascular mechanism (embolic, thrombotic, hemodynamic)
- Neuroimaging:
  - Head CT (noncontrast) if MRI is unavailable, mainly to exclude hemorrhage
  - CTA/MRA of the head and neck: Identify large vessel occlusions
  - MRI with diffusion-weighted imaging (DWI) is preferred to rule out infarction
  - Carotid Doppler ultrasound: Assess for carotid stenosis
- Cardiac workup:
  - ECG and Holter monitor: Detect atrial fibrillation
  - Echocardiography (TTE/TEE): Rule out cardiac embolic sources (e.g., PFO, LV thrombus)
- Laboratory tests:
  - Lipid panel and HbA1c: Evaluate for atherosclerosis risk
  - Hypercoagulability workup (in young patients or those without risk factors)
- Immediate management:
  - Admit high-risk patients (e.g., $ABCD^2$ score ≥4, atrial fibrillation, large vessel disease)
  - Aspirin (160–-25 mg) immediately, followed by dual antiplatelet therapy (DAPT) with aspirin + clopidogrel for 21–30 days if high risk
  - Blood pressure control: Maintain <140/90 mm Hg, but avoid aggressive lowering in acute phase
  - Statins (high intensity, e.g., atorvastatin 80 mg) for all patients with atherosclerosis
  - Anticoagulation for cardioembolic TIA (e.g., atrial fibrillation → DOAC/warfarin)
- Carotid intervention: Carotid endarterectomy (CEA) or carotid artery stenting (CAS) for symptomatic ≥50% carotid stenosis (CEA preferred in most cases)
- Long-term stroke prevention:
  - Lifestyle modifications: Smoking cessation, weight loss, and regular exercise. Mediterranean diet to improve vascular health
  - Blood pressure and lipid control: ACE inhibitors or ARBs preferred for hypertension. Statins for all patients with LDL >70 mg/dL

Nitin Agarwal
David T. Fernandes Cabral
Regan Shanahan

Thieme

Trigeminal Neuralgia (TGN)

Typical presentation includes electric-like pain sensation in the V2 and V3 distribution

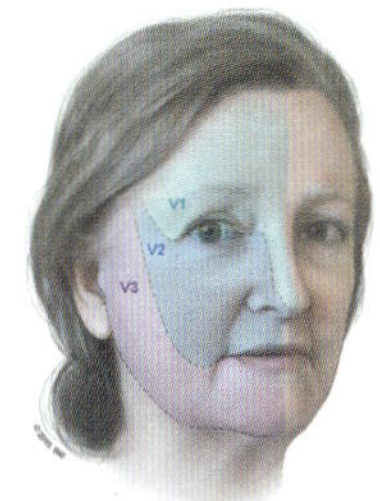

80–90% cases caused by neurovascular conflict

75% patients will fail medical therapy and require microvascular decompression

PRESENTATION

- Paroxysmal lancinating electric-like pain lasting a few seconds
- Triggered by sensory stimuli, confined to trigeminal branch distribution
- No neurological deficit
- Atypical presentation includes dull ache on the side of the face, hypersensitivity to touch

EPIDEMIOLOGY

- Age: typically, >50 years (average: 63 years)
- Laterality:
  - Right (60%)
  - Left (39%)
  - Both (1%)
- Divisions:
  - V1 (2%)
  - V2 (20%)
  - V3 (17%)
  - V1 & V2 (14%)
  - V2 & V3 (42%)
  - All three (5%)

PATHOPHYSIOLOGY

- Vascular compression of the trigeminal nerve at the root entry zone
  - 80% by the SCA, some AICA
  - Persistent primitive trigeminal artery
  - Dolichoectatic basilar artery
- Multiple Sclerosis within brainstem
- Posterior fossa tumor (rare)

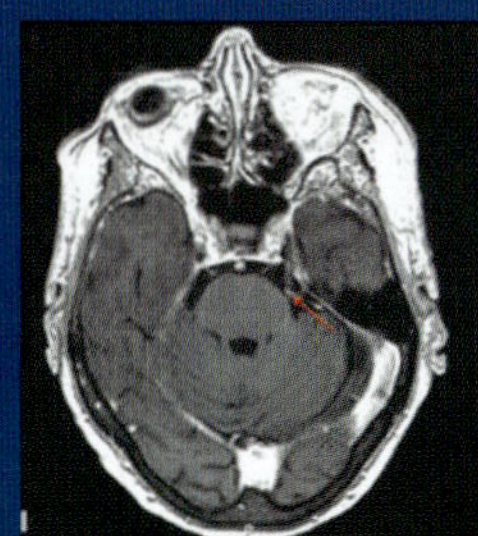

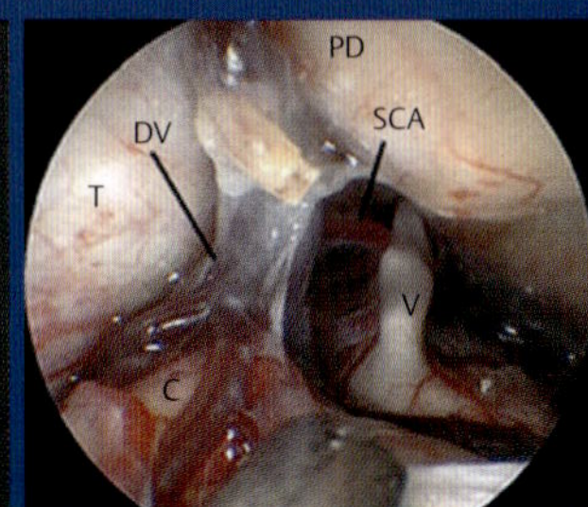

Left: MRI axial T1 image with contrast at the level of the midpons showing an aberrant loop of the superior cerebellar artery (red arrow) impinging on the root of the trigeminal nerve

Right: Endoscopic view approaching the trigeminal nerve for right-sided trigeminal neuralgia, with clear compression of the nerve by the superior cerebellar artery.
Abbreviations: C, cerebellum; DV, Dandy's vein; P, pons; PD, petrous dura; SCA, superior cerebellar artery; T, tentorium; V, fifth cranial nerve.

TREATMENTS

PHARMACOLOGICAL THERAPY

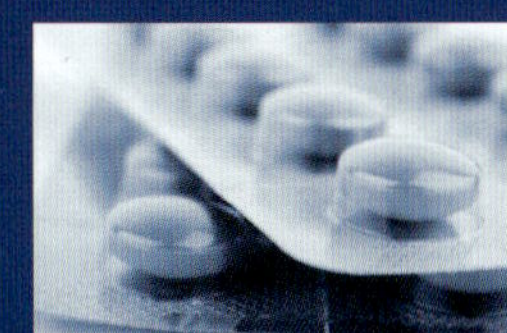

- Carbamazepine
- Oxcarbazepine
- Baclofen
- Gabapentin
- Botox injections
- Other antiepileptic agents

SURGICAL INTERVENTION

- Microvascular decompression
- Percutaneous trigeminal rhizotomy
- Percutaneous micro compression rhizolysis balloon
- Stereotactic radiosurgery in poor surgical candidates

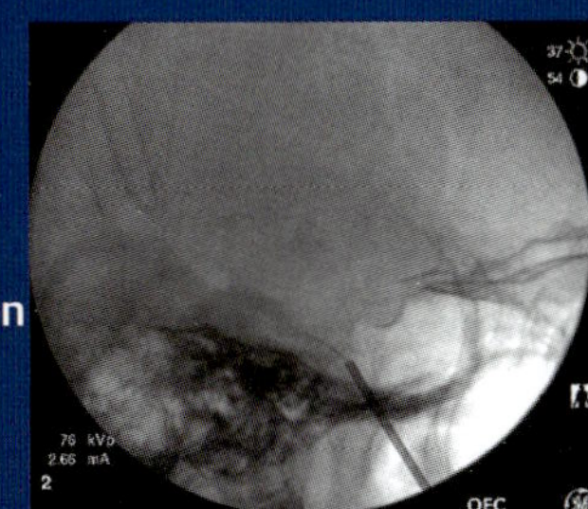

Percutaneous balloon rhizotomy for TGN

Further Reading

1. Tsementzis S ed. Trigeminal neuralgia. In: Differential Diagnosis in Neurology and Neurosurgery: A clinician's Pocket Guide 2nd ed. Noida: Thieme, 2019
2. Gagliardi F, Gragnaniello C, Mortini P, Caputy, A. eds. Intradural exposure. In: Operative Cranial Neurosurgical Anatomy 1st ed. Noida: Thieme; 2018

Nitin Agarwal
David T. Fernandes Cabral
Samuel Adida

Thieme

Tuberous Sclerosis (TSC)

Subependymal giant cell astrocytoma (SGCA) tumors is the most common neurosurgical indication among TSC patients

Genetics
- **Autosomal dominant**
- **Chromosome 9 TSC1 (Hamartin)**
- **Chromosome 16 TSC2 (Tuberin)**

Preoperative TTE needed to rule out cardiac rhabdomyomas

KEY FEATURES

- Neurocutaneous disorder characterized by the development of multiple benign tumors of the embryonic ectoderm (e.g., skin, eyes, and CNS)

CNS Manifestations
- Cortical/subcortical tubers
    - 50% in the frontal lobe
    - High T2 and low T1 with only 10% of tubers showing enhancement
    - Frequently calcify after two years of age
- Subependymal hamartomas
    - 88% associated with calcification, which is absent in early childhood
    - Visible within the first six months of age
    - Variable signal, frequently high T1 and iso to high T2
    - Enhancement is variable and not useful for distinguishing them from SGCA; only serial growth is reliable
- Subependymal giant cell astrocytoma (SGCA)
    - Peak occurrence at 8–18 years of age
    - Large and demonstrate growth
    - Intense enhancement
- White matter abnormalities
    - Variable appearance, with nodular, ill-defined, cystic and band-like lesions; radial bands thought to be relatively specific for TS

DIAGNOSIS

- Clinical triad
    - Seizures
    - Mental retardation
    - Sebaceous adenoma
- Infant: >3 "Ash leaf" macules with infantile myoclonus
- Older children/adults: generalized tonic-clonic or partial complex seizures and facial adenoma

DIAGNOSIS

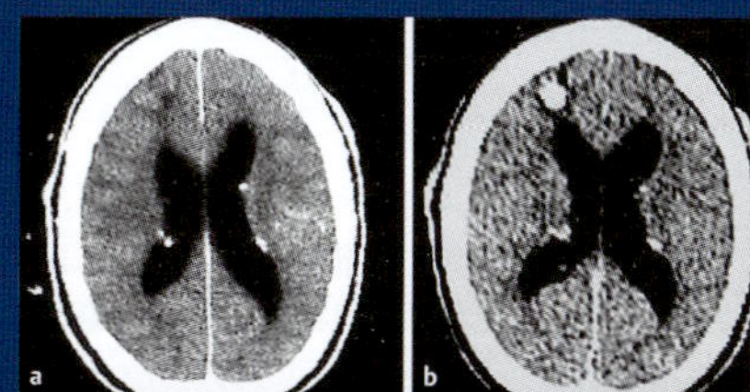

CT scans demonstrate multiple calcified tubers lining the lateral ventricles (candle guttering) and an enhancing right frontal tuber.

MANAGEMENT

Treatment dictated by individual manifestations
- Surgical resection of SGCAs
- Paraventricular tumors should be followed, removed only if they are symptomatic
- Infantile myoclonus may respond to steroids
- Seizures are treated with AEDs
- Surgery for intractable seizures may be considered when a seizure focus has been identified

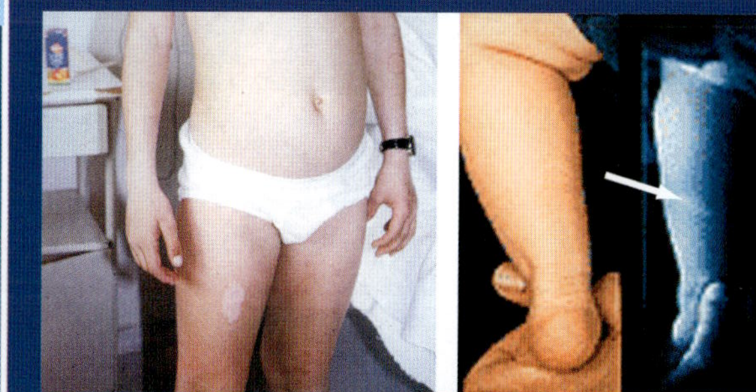

Further Reading
1. Citow JS, Macdonald RL, Puffer RC et al. eds. Comprehensive Neurosurgery Board Review 3rd ed. New York, NY: Thieme; 2019
2. Borsody M ed. Comprehensive Board Review in Neurology 1st ed. New York, NY: Thieme; 2007

Nitin Agarwal
David T. Fernandes Cabral
Samuel Adida

Thieme

Vertebrobasilar Insufficiency (VBI)-Part I

Signs and symptoms result from inadequate blood flow through the posterior cerebral circulation (vertebral arteries, basilar arteries, and their branches)

CLINICAL PRESENTATION

- VBI is inadequate blood flow through the posterior circulation of the brain and is a type of TIA
- The 5 Ds of VBI:
  - Drop attack: Sudden falls without loss of consciousness
  - Diplopia: Ischemia in the midbrain near ocular motor nuclei
  - Dysarthria: Ischemia in the lower brainstem
  - Defect (visual fields): Homonymous hemianopia (occipital ischemia)
    - Transient bilateral vision loss
  - Dizziness: Unexplained vertigo, often triggered by postural changes
- VBI is suspected if at least 2 of the following symptoms are present:
  - Bilateral motor/sensory symptoms
  - Diplopia
  - Dysarthria
  - Homonymous hemianopia
- VBI is suspected in patients with transient episodes of "dizziness" (vertigo that otherwise unexplained) that are initiated by positional changes
- VBI may sometimes be due to compression of VA at the C1–C2 level with:
  - Head turning
  - Os odontoideum: Rare anatomic variant in which the second cervical vertebra separates from the rest of the vertebra
  - Anterior atlantoaxial subluxation
  - Rotatory atlantoaxial subluxation

Further Readings
1. Meyers SP, ed. Differential Diagnosis in Neuroimaging: Spine. Stuttgart: Thieme Medical Publishers; 2016
2. Mattle H, Mumenthaler M, Taub E, eds. Fundamentals of Neurology: An Illustrated Guide. 2nd ed. Stuttgart: Thieme Medical Publishers; 2016

Nitin Agarwal
David T. Fernandes Cabral
Regan Shanahan

Thieme

Vertebrobasilar Insufficiency (VBI)-Part II

PATHOPHYSIOLOGY

- Atheromatous and stenotic lesions of the posterior circulation occur most frequently at the vertebral artery origin
- Symptoms may occur:
    - Hemodynamic insufficiency:
        - Subclavian steal
        - Stenosis of both vertebral arteries or of one where the other vessel is hypofunctional causing reduced distal flow in the face of inadequate collaterals
    - Embolism from ulcerations
    - Atherosclerotic occlusion of brainstem perforators
    - Vertebrobasilar hypoplasia

Feature	**VBI (posterior circulation TIA)**	**Hemispheric stroke (anterior circulation)**
Vascular territory	Vertebral & basilar arteries	Internal carotid, MCA, ACA
Onset	Transient (minutes to hours), recurrent	Acute, often persistent deficits
Motor deficits	Often bilateral or crossed (e.g., ipsilateral cranial nerve + contralateral limb weakness)	Contralateral hemiparesis (face, arm, leg based on MCA/ACA involvement)
Sensory deficits	Bilateral or asymmetric sensory loss	Contralateral hemisensory loss
Cranial nerve involvement	Diplopia, dysarthria, dysphagia, facial numbness, vertigo	Rarely affected unless large infarct
Cerebellar signs	Ataxia, dysmetria, nystagmus	Absent
Cortical signs (aphasia, neglect, gaze preference)	Rare	Common in MCA stroke
Vertigo & nausea	Frequent	Uncommon
Drop attacks	Can occur	Rare

Nitin Agarwal
David T. Fernandes Cabral
Regan Shanahan

Thieme

Vertebrobasilar Insufficiency (VBI)-Part III

Risk of stroke after first VBI-TIA has been estimated at 22% for the first year

EVALUATION & TREATMENT

- Evaluation: Four vessel angiography, sometimes with proactive maneuvers, CTA
- Bow hunter's stroke: Vertebrobasilar insufficiency caused by occlusion or stenosis of the vertebral artery associated with head movements
- Treatment:
    - Tissue plasminogen activator (tPA) can be used to treat ischemic vertebrobasilar (VB) strokes if administered within 4.5 h of symptom onset
    - Anticoagulation is the mainstay of medical management:
        - Alternatives include antiplatelets such as ASA
    - Endovascular treatment and stenting:
        - Angioplasty for basilar artery stenosis but not vertebral artery stroke
    - Surgical intervention:
        - Vertebral endarterectomy
        - Transposition of VA to ICA
        - Bypass grafting
        - C1–C2 posterior arthrodesis (may prevent life-threatening stroke for patients with os odontoideum)
        - ACDF:
            - Unroofing of the vertebral artery

Nitin Agarwal
David T. Fernandes Cabral
Regan Shanahan

Thieme

Vestibular Schwannomas

NF2-inactivating mutations in 50–75% of sporadic cases

Differential diagnosis includes meningiomas, epidermoid cysts, other schwannomas, cerebellar tumors, vascular lesions, and dural metastases

Observation and follow-up for asymptomatic or slowly growing tumors, radiosurgery for low Koos grade schwannomas or poor surgical candidates, and microsurgical resection for high Koos grade schwannomas with significant vestibulopathy or brainstem compression

PRESENTATION

- Vestibular schwannomas are benign and typically arise in the cerebellopontine angle. These tumors are usually solitary and sporadic, with onset around 40–50 years of age. They are a hallmark of NF2, and early or bilateral onset suggests a diagnosis of NF2
- Symptoms primarily result from compression of CNs, and include slowly progressive, high-frequency sensorineural hearing loss, vestibular dysfunction with nystagmus, cerebellar and brainstem compression, and increased ICP. In rare cases, palsies of CN V and CN XII may occur
- On T1 MRI, the tumor is iso- to mildly hypointense, with occasional cystic components. Post-contrast, it shows vivid enhancement. On T2 MRI, the tumor is hyperintense, and cystic components have high signal intensity. SWI may reveal blooming artifacts from microhemorrhages

RADIOGRAPHIC FEATURES

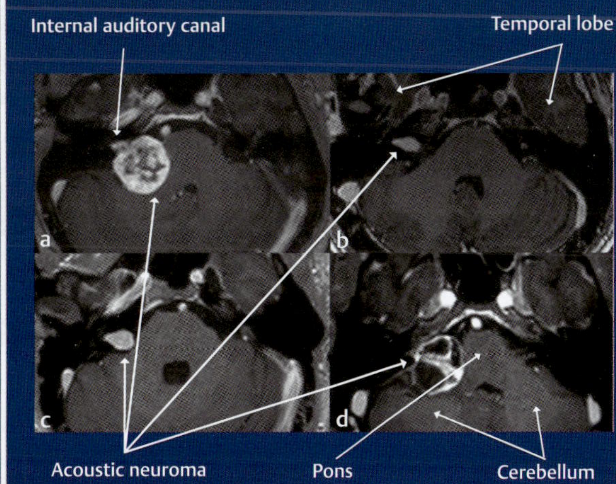

Representative images of different right-sided acoustic neuromas seen on MRI

TREATMENT

- The Koos classification of vestibular schwannomas stratifies tumors based on extrameatal extension and brainstem compression
- Observation is recommended for tumors <1.5 cm or intracanalicular, with serial imaging and audiograms. Natural history shows a 50% chance of hearing loss at 10 years with observation
- The 50/50 rule for serviceable hearing involves a pure tone audiogram threshold of <50 dB and a speech discrimination score >50%. Nonservicable hearing may permit aggressive treatment
- Stereotactic radiosurgery (SRS) can prevent tumor growth in small to medium-sized schwannomas (Koos grade I or II), achieving success rates >95% while preserving existing CN function. For larger or more complex tumors, such as those with significant cerebellar peduncle, brainstem, or fourth ventricle compression (Koos grade IV), surgery is recommended. Microsurgical resection remains the preferred treatment option for younger patients with minimal comorbidities

Further Reading

1. Greene J, Al-Dhahir MA. Acoustic Neuroma. StatPearls. Treasure Island, FL: StatPearls Publishing; 2024
2. Greenberg MS. Greenberg's Handbook of Neurosurgery. 10th ed. Stuttgart, Germany: Thieme Medical Publishing Group; 2023

Nitin Agarwal
David T. Fernandes Cabral
Samuel Adida

Thieme

Von Hippel-Lindau Syndrome

Von Hippel-Lindau (VHL) patients are neurosurgically managed for CNS hemiangioblastomas in the brain and spine.

Genetics
- Autosomal dominant
- VHL deletion
- Chromosome 3

Other tumor locations
- Endolymphatic sac
- Adrenal glands
- Pancreas
- Kidneys
- Epididymis
- Broad ligament

CNS FEATURES

- CNS hemangioblastoma (~70%)
  - Cerebellar (~60%)
    - Symptoms: Headache Vomiting, gait disturbances or ataxia
  - Spinal cord (~30%, commonly in cervical and thoracic spine)
    - Intradural
    - Symptoms: Pain, sensory and motor loss may develop with cord compression
  - Brain stem (~10%)
- Retinal hemangioblastoma (45–60%)
  - Most common presenting feature, vision loss in 35–55% of patients

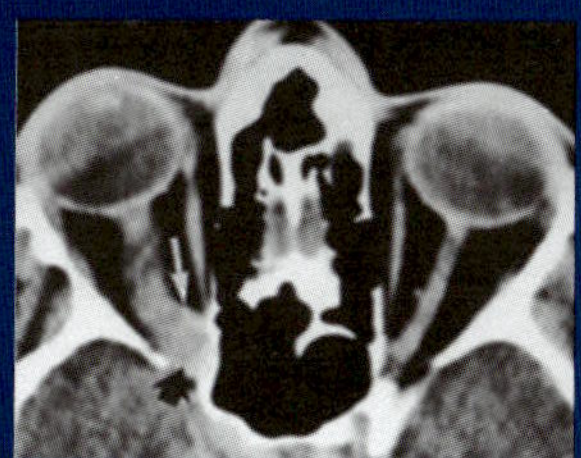

HEMANGIOBLASTOMA

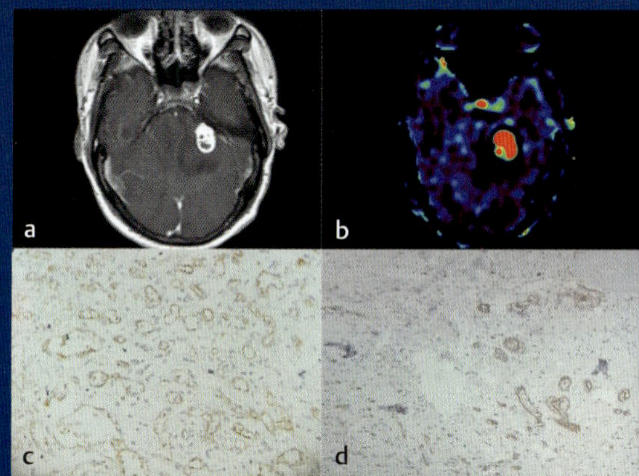

(a) Arterial spin labeling map; (b) Increased tumor blood flow; (c,d) Histopathological microvessel density

OTHER CONSIDERATIONS

- CNS hemangioblastoma is the main cause of death.
- Average life expectancy
  - 60 years for women
  - 67 years for men

SURGICAL INTERVENTION

- Surgical resection is first line treatment for hemangioblastoma
- Adjuvant radiotherapy may be used to reduce size and prevent growth

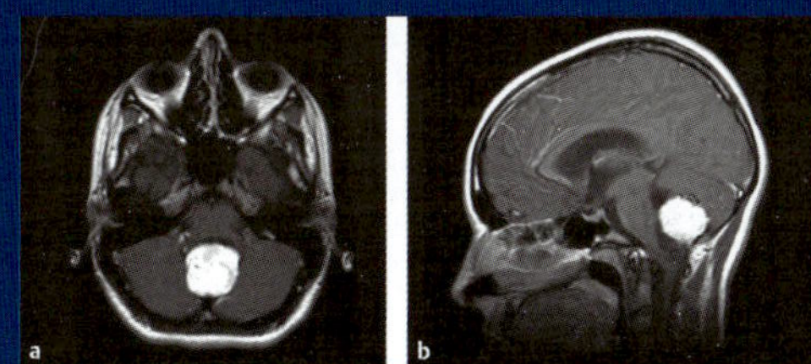

Further Reading
1. Catapano D, Muscarella LA, Guarnieri V et al. Hemangioblastomas of central nervous system: molecular genetic analysis and clinical management. Neurosurgery 2005;56(6):1215–1221
2. Lonser RR, Butman JA, Kiringoda R et al. Pituitary stalk hemangioblastomas in von Hippel-Lindau disease. J Neurosurg 2009;110(2):350–353

Nitin Agarwal
David T. Fernandes Cabral
Samuel Adida

Thieme

Spine

Ankylosing Spondylitis

- HLA-B27
- 90% male patients
- Seronegative RF

Radiographs are notable for “bamboo spine” appearance and fused SI joints

Associated symptoms:
- Uveitis
- Inflammatory bowel disease (IBD)
- Psoriasis
- Cardiovascular disease

PRESENTATION

- Back pain, morning pain/stiffness
- Reduced spinal mobility
  - Modified Schober’s test
  - FABER test
  - Lumbar side flexion
  - Occiput-to-wall distance
  - Chest expansion
- Extra-axial features
  - Oligoarthritis
  - Enthesitis of Achilles tendon

Age	< 40 years
Onset	Insidious
Activity	Relieves pain
Morning stiffness	Moderate >45 min
Inflammatory Markers	Elevated

RADIOGRAPHIC FEATURES

BAMBOO SPINE

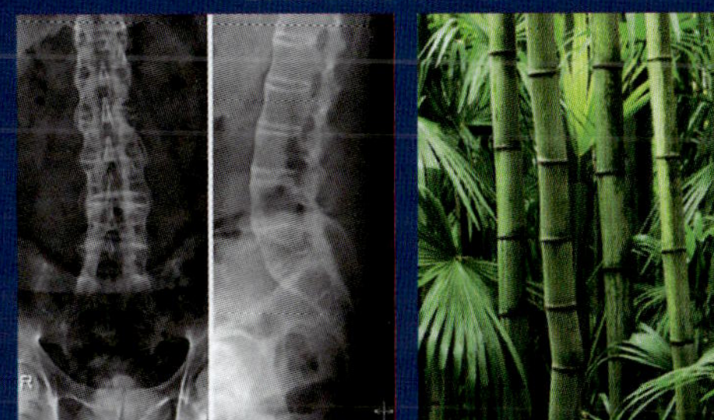

SACROILITIS

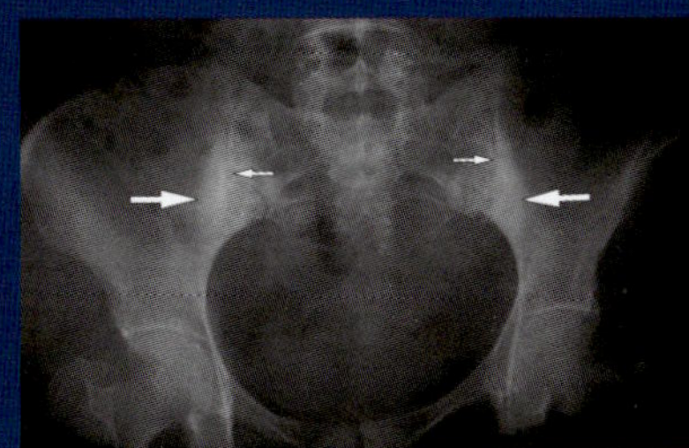

OTHER CONSIDERATIONS

COMPLICATIONS

- Limited mobility
- Osteoporosis
- Chalk stick fracture
- Restrictive lung disease
- Lung fibrosis
- Continued pain

PHARMACOLOGICAL THERAPY

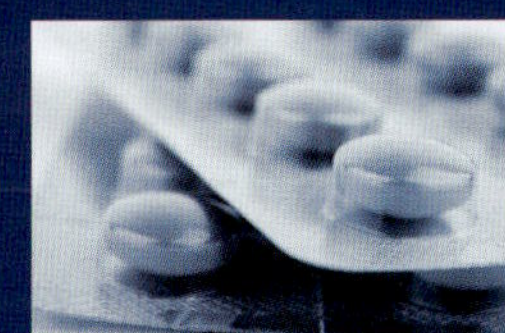

- NSAIDs
- Tumor necrosis inhibitor therapy
- Anti-interleukin-17 antibodies
- DMARDS

SURGICAL INTERVENTION

- Hip arthroplasty
  - Indication: Severe hip arthritis
- Spinal osteotomy
  - Indication: Severe kyphosis causing significant pain, physical disability, or psychological distress

Further Readings

1. Golder V, Schachna L. Ankylosing spondylitis: an update. Aust Fam Physician 2013;42(11):780–784.
2. Ward MM, Deodhar A, Gensler LS, et al. 2019 update of the American College of Rheumatology/Spondylitis Association of America/Spondyloarthritis Research and Treatment Network Recommendations for the treatment of ankylosing spondylitis and nonradiographic axial spondyloarthritis. Arthritis Rheumatol 2019;71(10):1599–1613

Nitin Agarwal
David T. Fernandes Cabral
Regan Shanahan

Thieme

Atlantoaxial Dislocation-Part I

Acute traumatic Atlantoaxial dislocation (AAD) with neurological deficits requires urgent decompression and stabilization, while chronic or congenital cases may be managed conservatively if asymptomatic or with surgical stabilization for severe deformities or instability

CLINICAL OVERVIEW

Introduction

- Atlantoaxial dislocation (AAD) refers to displacement of C1 (atlas) relative to C2 (axis), leading to significant craniocervical instability. AAD can result from traumatic or congenital causes, and if untreated, can lead to spinal cord compression and neurological deficits, including quadriplegia or death. It is a neurosurgical emergency requiring early identification and intervention

Classification

- AAD is typically classified based on the direction of dislocation and whether the transverse ligament is intact or disrupted
- Traumatic AAD (TAAD):
  - Mechanism: High-energy trauma (e.g., motor vehicle accidents, falls, or direct cervical trauma).
  - Pathophysiology:
  - Disruption of the transverse ligament, which normally stabilizes the C1–C2 complex
  - Displacement of the atlas (C1) relative to the axis (C2), which can either be anterior, posterior, or lateral
- Congenital AAD:
  - Down's syndrome (hypoplasia of the odontoid process, ligamentous laxity)
  - Rheumatoid arthritis (inflammatory destruction of the atlantoaxial joints)
  - Os odontoideum (a congenital defect in which the odontoid process is not fused to the C2 body)
  - Klippel–Feil syndrome (fusion of cervical vertebrae leading to instability)
- Types based on displacement:
  - Type I (anterior dislocation): Anterior displacement of C1 relative to C2, commonly from rupture of the transverse ligament
  - Type II (posterior dislocation): Rare, usually associated with severe traumatic injury or C1–C2 subluxation
  - Type III (rotatory dislocation): Characterized by lateral rotation of C1 relative to C2, often seen in Chiari malformation or rheumatoid arthritis

Nitin Agarwal
David T. Fernandes Cabral
Samuel Adida

Thieme

Atlantoaxial Dislocation-Part II

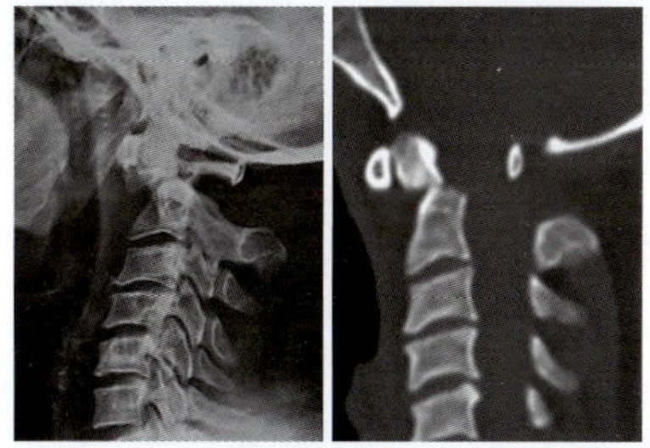

PRESENTATION & DIAGNOSIS

Presentation
- Neck pain, often with limited range of motion and spasm
- Neurological deficits
- Cervical myelopathy with progressive weakness, sensory loss, and bladder dysfunction
- Upper motor neuron signs (hyperreflexia, Babinski's sign) from spinal cord compression
- Severe cases: Quadriplegia and respiratory failure due to medullary compression
- Headaches, particularly occipital, from tension on the craniovertebral junction
- Torticollis (head tilt or twisting) in rotatory dislocations

Imaging
- X-ray (AP and lateral cervical spine):
    - ADI (atlanto-dens interval): Normal ADI is <3 mm in adults and <5 mm in children. An increased ADI indicates ligamentous disruption and dislocation
    - Open-mouth odontoid view: Look for overhang of the lateral masses of C1 relative to C2, indicating dislocation
    - Lateral X-ray: Assess C1–C2 alignment and look for anterior or posterior displacement of the atlas
- Cervical spine CT (gold standard):
    - Essential for detailed visualization of bone structures, C1–C2 alignment, and transverse ligament integrity
    - Fracture of the odontoid or atlas may be present in traumatic cases
    - Can evaluate for associated injuries like vertebral artery injury or fracture
- Cervical spine MRI: Critical for assessing spinal cord compression:
    - Evaluate the transverse ligament (MRI may show disruption or thickening)
    - Evaluate for associated neurological deficits, such as spinal cord edema
- CT angiography for suspected vascular injury

Nitin Agarwal
David T. Fernandes Cabral
Samuel Adida

Thieme

Atlantoaxial Dislocation-Part III

AAD is often a result of trauma or congenital conditions, with the most common cause being rupture of the transverse ligament leading to C1–C2 instability

MANAGEMENT

- The choice between posterior C1–C2 fusion (Goel–Harms or Magerl's technique) and anterior odontoid screw fixation depends on the fracture type, alignment, and patient anatomy. Posterior fusion is preferred for most traumatic dislocations due to its ability to stabilize both the atlantoaxial joint and cervical spine, while anterior fusion may be more appropriate for isolated odontoid fractures or certain congenital cases

Acute TAAD
- Emergency decompression is required if there are neurological deficits or spinal cord compression
- Initial immobilization with a halo vest or rigid cervical collar to prevent further damage
- Surgical management:
- C1–C2 fusion (posterior fusion or anterior odontoid screw fixation) to provide stability and prevent further dislocation
- Anterior C1–C2 fixation if the posterior approach is not feasible
- Decompression if there is significant cord compression

Congenital or Chronic AAD
- Conservative management with a rigid collar or halo vest may be sufficient in stable cases with no neurological deficits
- Surgical intervention:
    - Posterior C1–C2 fusion with or without occipitocervical fusion for patients with congenital instability or associated conditions (e.g., Down's syndrome, rheumatoid arthritis)
    - Occiput–C2 fusion in patients with severe deformity or craniocervical instability

Nitin Agarwal
David T. Fernandes Cabral
Samuel Adida

Thieme

C1 (Atlas) Fracture-Part I

Jefferson's fractures (C1 burst fractures) result from axial loading and are unstable if transverse ligament disruption occurs, requiring MRI assessment and possible surgical stabilization

CLINICAL OVERVIEW

Introduction

- C1 fractures involve the atlas, the ring-like first cervical vertebra, which articulates with the occipital condyles and C2 (axis) to provide head motion
- These fractures often result from axial loading injuries (e.g., diving, high-impact trauma) and are frequently associated with C2 fractures (especially type II odontoid fractures) and craniocervical instability

Classification

- Jefferson's fracture (burst fracture):
    - Classic four-part fracture involving the anterior and posterior arches due to axial compression
    - Often unstable if transverse ligament is disrupted, leading to atlantoaxial instability
    - Mechanism: High-energy axial loading (e.g., diving headfirst into shallow water)
- Posterior arch fracture:
    - Most common isolated C1 fracture (~50%), occurring from forced hyperextension
    - Stable injury, as the ring remains intact
- Lateral mass fracture:
    - Usually results from shearing forces; often unstable, requiring careful evaluation of craniocervical alignment
- Transverse ligament disruption (atlantoaxial instability):
    - Key determinant of stability in C1 fractures
    - If the transverse ligament is disrupted (>5 mm ADI on flexion–extension X-rays or MRI), surgical stabilization is required

Nitin Agarwal
David T. Fernandes Cabral
Samuel Adida

Thieme

C1 (Atlas) Fracture-Part II

CT is the gold standard for diagnosis, but MRI is critical for evaluating transverse ligament integrity, which dictates management (conservative vs. surgical)

PRESENTATION & DIAGNOSIS

Presentation
- Neck pain and stiffness, often without neurological deficits (spinal canal is wide at C1)
- Occipital neuralgia due to irritation of the C2 nerve roots
- Neurologic deficits are rare unless there is associated spinal cord injury (high-impact trauma, craniocervical instability)
- Concomitant injuries common (~50%): C2 fractures, traumatic brain injury (TBI), or vascular injury (vertebral artery dissection)

Imaging
- CT cervical spine (gold standard):
  - Best for fracture characterization (Jefferson, posterior arch, lateral mass)
  - Look for overhang of lateral masses (>6.9 mm total on AP open-mouth view = transverse ligament rupture, unstable fracture)
- MRI cervical spine:
  - Essential for assessing transverse ligament integrity (disruption = instability)
  - Identifies ligamentous injuries and spinal cord involvement
- X-rays (open-mouth odontoid view):
  - Jefferson's fracture: Lateral mass overhang
  - Atlanto-dens interval (ADI >3 mm in adults, >5 mm in children) suggests transverse ligament disruption

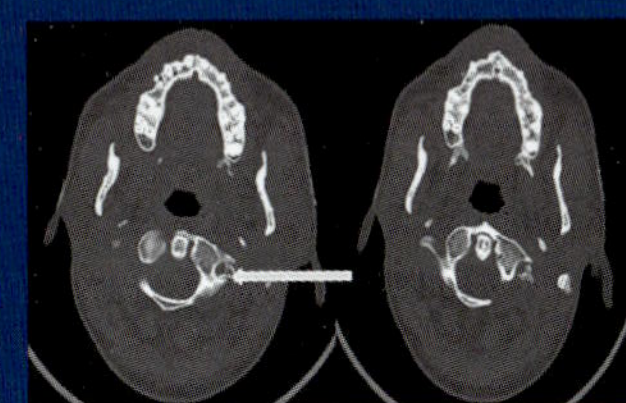

Axial images of CT of the cervical spine showing fracture of the atlas with involvement of the transverse process with inward and medial displacement (*arrow*)

Nitin Agarwal
David T. Fernandes Cabral
Samuel Adida

Thieme

C1 (Atlas) Fracture-Part III

Stable fractures can be managed with rigid immobilization (e.g., cervical collar or halo), while unstable fractures require C1–C2 or occipitocervical fusion to prevent craniocervical instability

MANAGEMENT

Stable Fractures (Intact Transverse Ligament, No Overhang >6.9 mm)

- Rigid cervical orthosis (Miami J, Aspen) or halo vest immobilization for 8–12 weeks
- Serial imaging to monitor healing

Unstable Fractures (Transverse Ligament Rupture, Craniocervical Instability)

- Definitive surgical stabilization:
  - C1–C2 fusion (Goel–Harms or Magerl's technique) for atlantoaxial instability
  - Occiput–C2 fusion if occipitocervical instability is present

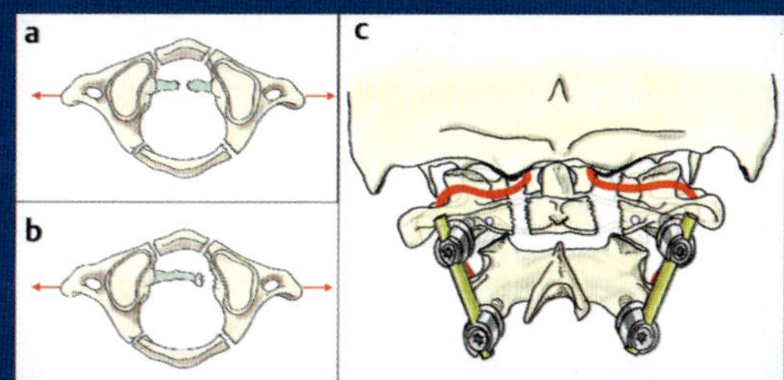

Schematic diagram showing Gehweiler type 3B type 1 (a) and 3B type 2 (b) fractures showing disruption of the transverse atlantal ligament in the latter. (c) The C1–C2 lateral mass and screw fixation of type 3 fractures highlighting the lateral than usual trajectory (*violet circles*) needed for C1 lateral mass screws

Nitin Agarwal
David T. Fernandes Cabral
Samuel Adida

Thieme

C2 (Axis) Fracture-Part I

C2 fractures are classified into odontoid (dens) fractures and hangman's fractures, with type II odontoid fractures being the most common and unstable due to high nonunion risk

CLINICAL OVERVIEW

Introduction

- C2 fractures involve the axis, the second cervical vertebra, which plays a critical role in atlantoaxial stability and rotational motion. These fractures commonly result from high-energy trauma (MVAs, falls, diving injuries) and can range from stable to highly unstable patterns. The two most clinically relevant C2 fractures are odontoid fractures (dens fractures) and hangman's fractures

Classification

- Odontoid fractures (dens fractures)—Anderson and D'Alonzo classification:
    - Type I: Fracture of the upper dens tip (rare, usually stable)
    - Type II: Fracture at the base of the dens, at the junction with the C2 body (most common and most unstable due to poor vascular supply, high nonunion risk)
    - Type III: Fracture extending into the C2 vertebral body, often stable, with good healing potential
- Hangman's fracture (traumatic spondylolisthesis of C2)—Levine and Edwards classification:
    - Type I: Nondisplaced fracture of the bilateral C2 pars interarticularis; stable
    - Type II: Displaced fracture with C2–C3 disk disruption, often unstable
    - Type IIA: Severe angulation without translation; highly unstable due to ligamentous injury
    - Type III: C2 pars fracture with facet dislocation; highly unstable
- Other C2 fractures:
    - C2 body fractures: Result from axial loading and are often stable unless associated with ligamentous injury
    - C2 lateral mass fractures: Typically from flexion–compression mechanisms; stability depends on associated injuries

Nitin Agarwal
David T. Fernandes Cabral
Samuel Adida

Thieme

C2 (Axis) Fracture-Part II

In elderly patients, type II odontoid fractures are more common and often present with subtle symptoms due to lower-energy mechanisms (e.g., falls)

PRESENTATION & DIAGNOSIS

Presentation
- Neck pain and limited range of motion (often severe)
- Neurological deficits are uncommon unless associated with spinal cord injury (high-energy trauma, severe displacement)
- High risk of vertebral artery injury in displaced fractures
- Odontoid fractures in the elderly ("low-energy ground-level falls") can present subtly but have high mortality

Imaging
- CT of the cervical spine (gold standard): Defines fracture morphology, displacement, and C1–C2 instability
- MRI of the cervical spine: Critical for assessing ligamentous injury, spinal cord involvement, and ruling out transverse ligament disruption (if atlantoaxial instability is suspected)
- X-ray (AP, lateral, open-mouth odontoid view):
    - Odontoid fractures: Look for dens displacement and prevertebral swelling
    - Hangman's fracture: Look for C2 anterolisthesis over C3, widened C2–C3 disk space

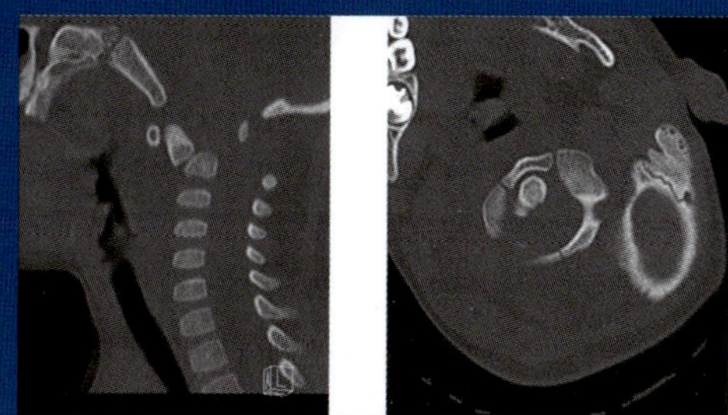

Sagittal (left) and axial (right) view CT without contrast of the cervical spine, revealing grade IV anterolisthesis of the dens due to a type II dens fracture

Nitin Agarwal
David T. Fernandes Cabral
Samuel Adida

Thieme

C2 (Axis) Fracture-Part III

Management is dictated by fracture stability, with stable fractures treated conservatively (rigid collar or halo) and unstable fractures requiring surgical fixation (C1–C2 fusion or anterior odontoid screw for odontoid fractures, C2–C3 fusion for unstable hangman's fractures)

MANAGEMENT

Odontoid Fractures
- Type I: Conservative (rigid cervical collar for 6–8 weeks)
- Type II: <5 mm displacement, intact transverse ligament → Halo or rigid collar for 8–12 weeks
- >5 mm displacement, nonunion risk (elderly), or angulation >10 degrees → Surgical fixation (C1–C2 posterior fusion or anterior odontoid screw fixation)
- Type III: Typically heals with rigid immobilization (Miami J, C2–C3 fusion for instability and facet dislocationAspen, or Halo)

Hangman's Fracture
- Type I: Rigid cervical collar (6–8 weeks)
- Types II and IIA: Halo immobilization or C2–C3 anterior fusion if unstable
- Type III: Posterior

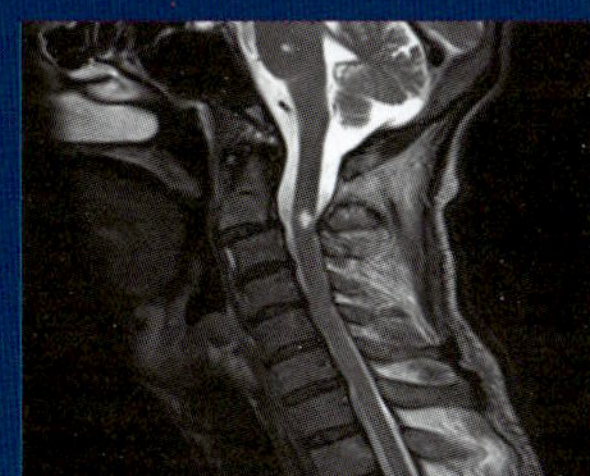

Magnetic resonance imaging showing cord signal change at C2–C3 disk space level with anterolisthesis and retroangulation of the C2 body

Nitin Agarwal
David T. Fernandes Cabral
Samuel Adida

Thieme

Cervical Spine-Part I

C5–C6 and C6–C7 are common sites for herniated disks and spondylotic myelopathy due to their high range of motion and load-bearing roles

ANATOMY

Key vertebrae:
- C1 (atlas): Unique ring-shaped vertebra with no body or spinous process:
    - Articulates with the occipital condyles, allowing flexion and extension ("yes" motion)
    - Important landmarks: anterior and posterior arches, lateral masses
- C2 (axis): Features the dens (odontoid process), a pivot point for rotation of the atlas ("no" motion):
    - Stabilized by the transverse ligament
- C7 (vertebra prominence): The most prominent spinous process, easily palpable; transition point between the cervical and thoracic spine

Joints:
- Atlanto-occipital joint (C0–C1): Primarily flexion/extension
- Atlantoaxial joint (C1–C2): Allows rotational movement
- Intervertebral joints: Facilitate flexion, extension, lateral bending, and limited rotation
- Ligaments:
    - Cruciate ligament complex (transverse and alar ligaments): Stabilizes C1 and C2
    - Anterior and posterior longitudinal ligaments: Run the length of the spine, providing stability
    - Ligamentum flavum: Connects adjacent laminae, preserving spinal canal integrity
- Foramina:
    - Transverse foramina in C1–C6 transmit the vertebral arteries

Nitin Agarwal
David T. Fernandes Cabral
Samuel Adida

Thieme

Cervical Spine-Part II

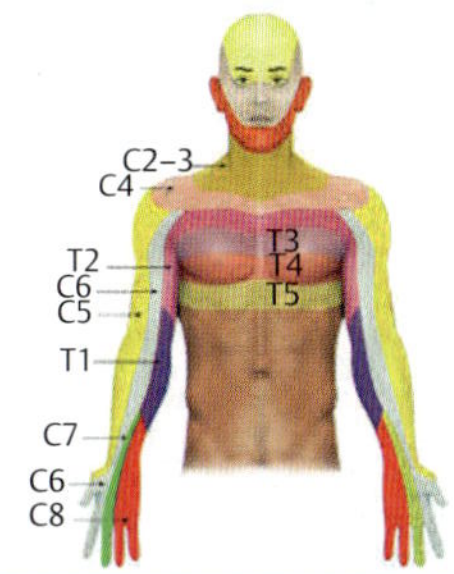

Cervical dermatomes

PHYSICAL EXAMINATION

- Observe the neck for alignment, swelling, muscle atrophy, or visible deformities
- Palpate the spinous processes from C2 to C7 for tenderness or step-offs (e.g., in trauma)
- Assess paraspinal and trapezius muscles for spasm or asymmetry
- Palpate the occiput and suboccipital region for tenderness (e.g., cervicogenic headache)
- Range of motion
- Motor testing (myotomes):
    - C5: Shoulder abduction (deltoid)
    - C6: Elbow flexion, wrist extension
    - C7: Elbow extension, wrist flexion
    - C8: Finger flexion
    - T1: Finger abduction
- Sensory testing (dermatomes):
    - C5: Lateral shoulder
    - C6: Lateral forearm and thumb
    - C7: Middle finger
    - C8: Little finger
    - T1: Medial forearm
- Reflexes:
    - C5: Biceps tendon
    - C6: Brachioradialis tendon
    - C7: Triceps tendon
- Spurling's test: Axial compression with neck extension and rotation to assess for radiculopathy (positive if pain radiates down the arm)
- Lhermitte's sign: Neck flexion causing an electric shock sensation may indicate cervical myelopathy
- Distraction test: Relieves radicular pain, suggesting nerve root compression

Nitin Agarwal
David T. Fernandes Cabral
Samuel Adida

Thieme

Cervical Spine-Part III

The transverse ligament of the atlas is essential for stabilizing the dens (C2) and preventing atlantoaxial subluxation, which can cause spinal cord compression

PATHOLOGY & MANAGEMENT

Pathology:
- Degenerative disease: Commonly affects the C5–C6 and C6–C7 levels due to high mobility and load bearing.
- Trauma: Common injuries include Jefferson fractures (C1), odontoid fractures (C2), and hangman's fractures (C2 pedicle)
- Stenosis: May lead to myelopathy, presenting with upper motor neuron signs
- Herniated Disk: Can cause radiculopathy or myelopathy depending on the level of compression

Clinical imaging:
- X-ray: Initial assessment; lateral view identifies alignment, fractures, and prevertebral soft tissue swelling
- CT scan: Preferred for bony detail and trauma
- MRI: Gold standard for soft tissue, spinal cord, and nerve root evaluation

Surgical considerations:
- Anterior approaches (ACDF): Effective for disk herniations and spondylotic myelopathy
- Posterior approaches: Indicated for laminectomies with or without instrumented fusion
- Craniovertebral junction stabilization: Requires detailed knowledge of C1–C2 anatomy and ligaments

Nitin Agarwal
David T. Fernandes Cabral
Samuel Adida

Thieme

Chondromyxoid Fibromas

<1%
of all spinal tumors

Histological features include:
- Lobular arrangement of scattered tumor cells with spindled or stellate nuclei
- Cartilage-like lacunae and microcysts containing chondromyxoid material

ETIOLOGY

- Chondromyxoid fibroma is a rare benign tumor of cartilaginous origin
- They account for less than 0.5% of all bone tumors, and 8% of all chondromyxoid fibromas are of vertebral origin

PRESENTATION

- Signs and symptoms of spinal cord or nerve root compression:
    - Localized back or neck pain
    - Radicular pain
    - Sensory and motor deficits
    - Bladder and bowel dysfunction
    - Gait disturbances

HISTOLOGIC FEATURES

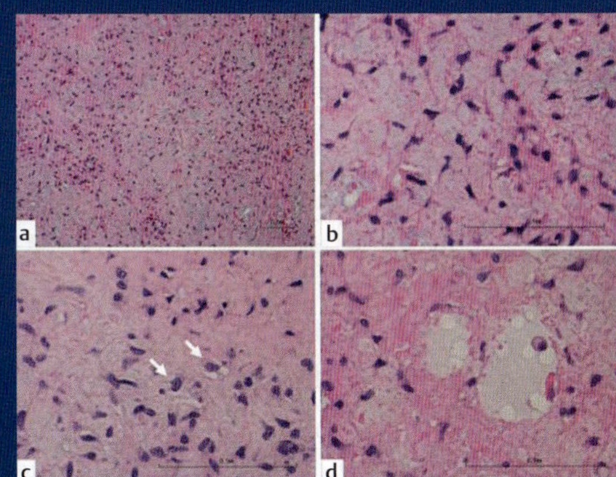

Chondromyxoid fibroma displays a lobular or zonal arrangement of (a) scattered tumor cells with (b) spindled or stellate nuclei. Small foci of tumor cells that (c) resemble cartilage lacunae and (d) microcysts containing chondromyxoid material can be observed

OTHER CONSIDERATIONS

- Chondromyxoid fibroma tends to be a slow-growing osteolytic lesion that erodes cortical bone
- Diseases that must be differentiated from chondromyxoid fibroma include chondrosarcoma, enchondroma, and chondroblastoma. Of note, chondromyxoid fibroma stains positive for S-100

TREATMENT

- Simple curettage without filling the defect can lead to recurrence rates ranging from 20 to 80%. Curettage with bone grafting or cement fixation has a lower recurrence rate of approximately 7%

Further Reading
1. Li C, Li S, Hu W. Chondromyxoid fibroma of the cervical spine: a case report. World J Clin Cases 2022;10(17):5748–5755
2. Zillmer DA, Dorfman HD. Chondromyxoid fibroma of bone: thirty-six cases with clinicopathologic correlation. Hum Pathol 1989;20:952–964
3. Basak B, Haragan A, Shackcloth M, Thekkudan J. Chondromyxoid fibroma of the rib: a rare benign tumor with potential for local recurrence. Cureus 2021;13:e19172

Nitin Agarwal
David T. Fernandes Cabral
Samuel Adida

Thieme

Desmoid Fibromas

Genetic risk factors include mutations in APC, seen in familial adenomatous polyposis (FAP) and CTNNB1, which affects the Wnt/β-catenin signaling pathway

Gardner syndrome is a variant of FAP that may present with extraintestinal manifestations, including desmoid fibromas

Surgical management aims for complete excision; however, when infeasible, subtotal resection with radiotherapy may be performed

PRESENTATION

- Desmoid fibroma is a rare neoplasm of bone, accounting for less than 0.1% of all bone tumors and 0.3% of benign bone tumors
- Despite being a slow-growing and benign tumor, desmoid fibroma exhibits locally aggressive and infiltrative growth, which can result in significant clinical symptoms
- Patients may present with signs and symptoms related to spinal cord or nerve root compression, including localized back or neck pain, radicular pain, sensory and motor deficits, bladder and bowel dysfunction, and gait ataxia
- These symptoms can overlap with a wide range of differential diagnoses, such as giant cell tumors, unicameral and aneurysmal bone cysts, fibrous dysplasia, osteosarcoma, and metastases

RADIOGRAPHIC FEATURES

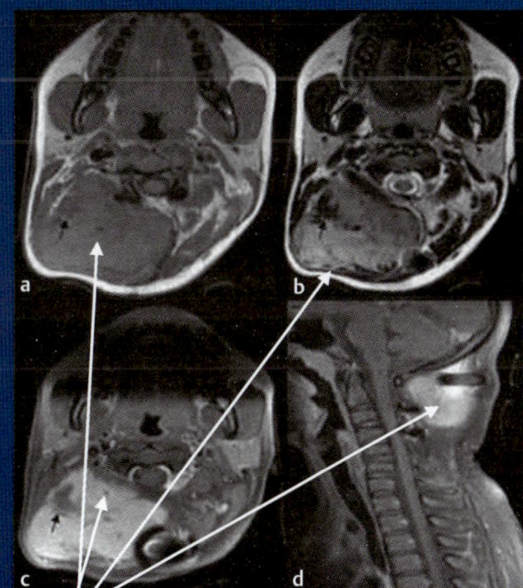

T1-weighted (a, c, d) and T2-weighted (b) MRI images of a desmoid fibroma extending from C1 to C4 posteriorly

HISTOLOGY

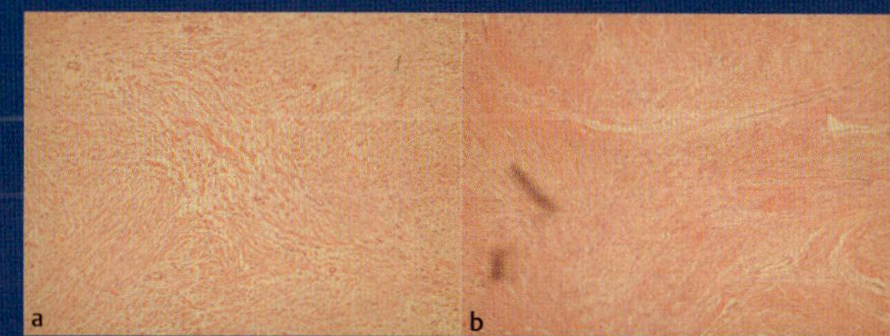

Histology shows cells with pale eosinophilic cytoplasm and spindle-shaped morphology (a), and collagen with keloidal features (b)

TREATMENT

- Radical resection is the first-line treatment, as incomplete excision leads to high rates of recurrence
- If complete resection is not feasible, subtotal excision combined with postoperative RT is an alternative. In cases involving the spine, decompressive laminectomy can be performed

Further Reading

1. Yin H, Zhang D, Wu Z. et al. Desmoplastic fibroma of the spine: a series of 12 cases and outcomes. Spine J 2014;14(8):1622–1628

Nitin Agarwal
David T. Fernandes Cabral
Samuel Adida

Thieme

Ewing's Sarcomas

<1%
of all spinal tumors

Genetic risk
t(11;22)

Male > Female

ETIOLOGY

- Ewing's sarcoma is a neuroectodermal tumor most commonly occurring in the first or second decade of life. The diagnosis is based on histology, with the tumor expressing CD99 and a characteristic t(11;22) translocation on chromosome 22
- Although Ewing's sarcoma is primarily a malignant bone tumor that commonly affects the appendicular skeleton, involvement of the axial skeleton and spine is rare
- Symptoms of spinal cord or nerve root compression may include localized back or neck pain, radicular pain, sensory and motor deficits, bladder and bowel dysfunction, and gait disturbances

RADIOGRAPHIC FEATURES

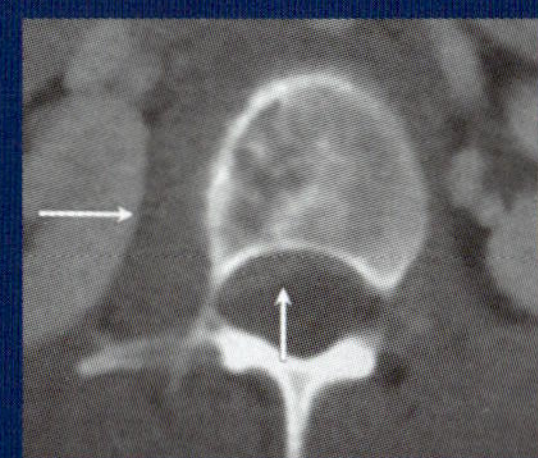

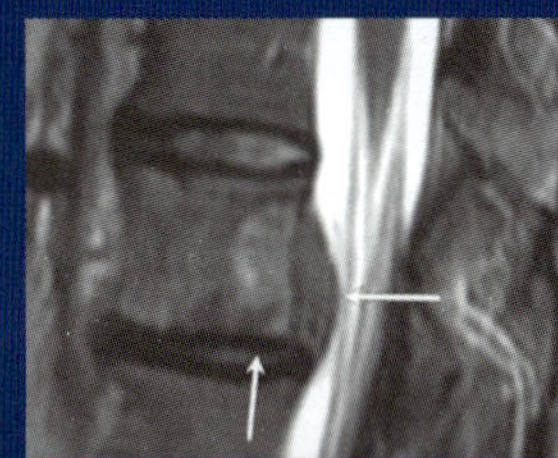

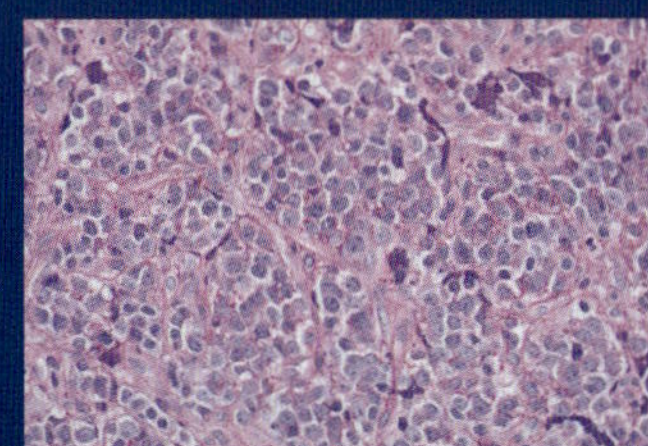

CT and T2 MRI reveal Ewing's sarcoma involving the right lumbar vertebral body. Histologically, sheets and nests of primitive-appearing round, blue cells can be seen

X-ray/CT
- Sclerosis, "sunburst" or spiculated periosteal reaction, and cystic components

MRI
- T1: Low to intermediate signal
- T1 with contrast: Heterogeneous signal, prominent enhancement
- T2: Heterogeneous signal, hair-on-end low-signal striations

Nuclear medicine bone scan
- Uptake of Gallium^{67} and Technetium^{99m}

TREATMENT

- Laminectomy is often used for circumferential cord compression. Neoadjuvant chemotherapy shrinks the tumor, improves survival, and aids resection. Postoperative chemotherapy and radiation control micrometastases. Primary radiotherapy is avoided due to the risk of worsening neural compression

Further Reading
1. Ansari MN, Gupta A, Jain DK et al. The Ewing's sarcoma of cervical spine: a rare occurrence. Spinal Cord Ser Cases 2022;8(1):68
2. Cherraqi A, Lemrabet A, Dokal ID et al. Primary Ewing's sarcoma of the spine: about a case. Glob Pediatr Health 2022;9:2333794X221123874.
3. Greenberg MS. Greenberg's Handbook of Neurosurgery. 10th ed. Stuttgart, Germany: Thieme Medical Publishing Group; 2023

Nitin Agarwal
David T. Fernandes Cabral
Samuel Adida

Thieme

Extradural Spinal Tumors

60%

of all spinal tumors

Primary extradural spinal cancers:

Giant cell tumor, hemangioma, osteoblastoma, osteochondroma, osteoid osteoma, chordoma, chondrosarcoma, Ewing's sarcoma, osteosarcoma, lymphoma, and multiple myeloma

Extradural spinal metastases:

Most commonly from breast, lung, prostate, kidney, and gastrointestinal primary cancers

PRESENTATION

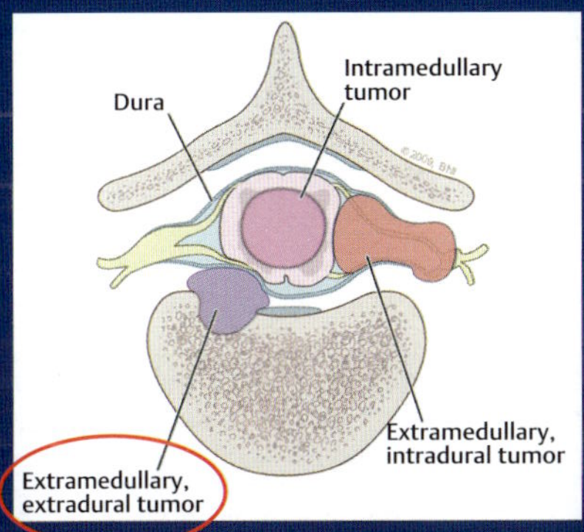

- Spinal tumors are classified as extradural, intradural extramedullary, or intradural intramedullary. Extradural tumors are most commonly metastases and may cause intractable pain, neural deficits, and spinal instability
- Signs and symptoms of spinal cord or nerve root compression include localized back or neck pain, radicular pain, sensory and motor deficits, bladder and bowel dysfunction, and gait disturbances

RADIOGRAPHIC FEATURES

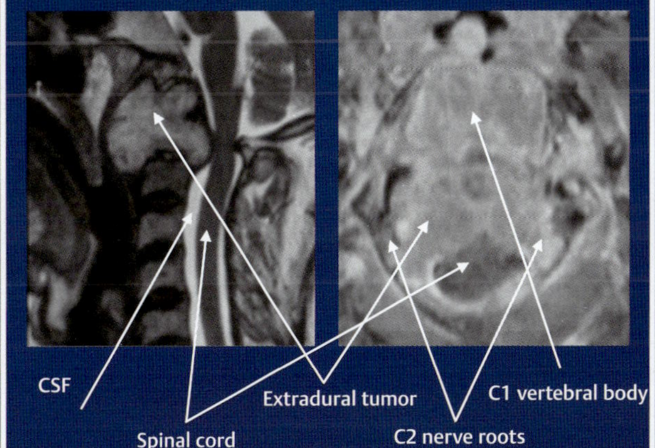

T2 MRI of thyroid carcinoma metastases to the C1 and C2 vertebral bodies shows compression of the spinal cord and nerve roots, making it difficult to appreciate the anatomy in the axial plane

TREATMENT

- The NOMS decision framework is used to facilitate decision-making in the treatment of spinal metastases
- Treatment for patients with spinal metastases is palliative and focuses on decompressing the spinal cord, providing mechanical stability, and achieving local tumor control
- Surgical options include laminectomy with tumor resection and corpectomy, as well as instrumented reconstruction of the spine. Cement augmentation of involved vertebrae with vertebroplasty or kyphoplasty may also be an option
- Radiotherapy and radiosurgery can prevent tumor growth and reduce the morbidity associated with open surgery

Further Reading

1. Zhao Y, Liu F, Wang W. Treatment progress of spinal metastatic cancer: a powerful tool for improving the quality of life of the patients. J Orthop Surg Res 2023;18(1):563

Nitin Agarwal
David T. Fernandes Cabral
Samuel Adida

Thieme

Intradural Extramedullary Tumors

Genetic risk
NF 1*, *NF 2*, and *VHL

Common tumors and their derivatives:

- **Schwannomas (Schwann cells)**
- **Neurofibromas (Schwann cells, fibroblasts, and nerve fibers)**
- **Meningiomas (arachnoid cap cells)**
- **Hemangioblastomas (endothelial and stromal cells)**
- **Other common tumors include ependymomas, peripheral nerve sheath tumors, and paragangliomas**
- **Leptomeningeal metastases are rare**

PRESENTATION

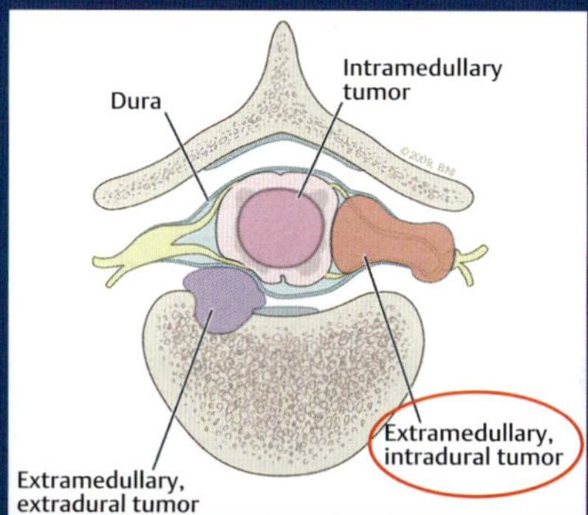

- Spinal tumors are classified as extradural, intradural extramedullary, or intradural intramedullary. Intradural extramedullary tumors are typically benign and located within the dural sac, but outside the spinal cord
- Spinal cord or nerve root compression may present with localized back or neck pain, radicular pain, sensory and motor deficits, bladder and bowel dysfunction, and gait disturbances

RADIOGRAPHIC FEATURES

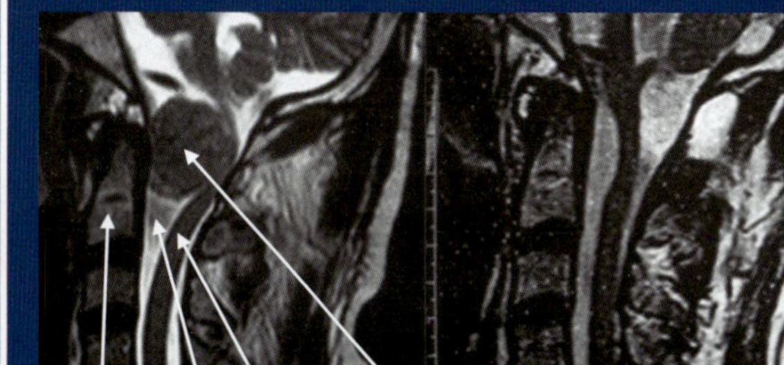

T2 MRI of a homogenously enhancing cervical meningioma, both prior to and after surgical resection

TREATMENT

- Factors that affect treatment options:
  - Tumor size
  - Tumor location
  - Tumor growth rate
  - Candidacy for surgery
- Conservative treatment:
  - For asymptomatic and small tumors
  - Monitor growth with serial imaging
- Surgical treatment:
  - For symptomatic and/or large tumors
  - Surgical resection is preferable
  - Radiation therapy and stereotactic radiosurgery are effective but should not be considered substitutes for complete removal

Further Reading

1. Ogden A. Treatment Options for Intradural Extramedullary Tumors. Neurosurgeons of New Jersey. Accessed March 22, 2022 at: https://www.neurosurgeonsofnewjersey.com/blog/intradural-extramedullary-tumors/
2. Arnautovic K, Arnautovic A et al. Extramedullary intradural spinal tumors: a review of modern diagnostic and treatment options and a report of a series. Bosn J Basic Med Sci 2009;9(Suppl 1):S40–S45
3. Cofano F, Giambra C, Costa P et al. Management of extramedullary intradural spinal tumors: the impact of clinical status, intraoperative neurophysiological monitoring and surgical approach on outcomes in a 12-year double-center experience. Front Neurol 2020;11:598619

Nitin Agarwal
David T. Fernandes Cabral
Samuel Adida

Thieme

Intradural Intramedullary Spinal Tumors

2–5%
of all spinal tumors

Genetic risk
NF 1*, *NF 2*, and *VHL

Common tumors and their derivatives:

- **Ependymomas (ependymal cells)**
- **Astrocytomas (astrocytes)**
- **Hemangioblastomas (endothelial and stromal cells)**
- **Other common tumors include lipomas, germ cell tumors, gangliogliomas, lymphomas, and metastases**

PRESENTATION

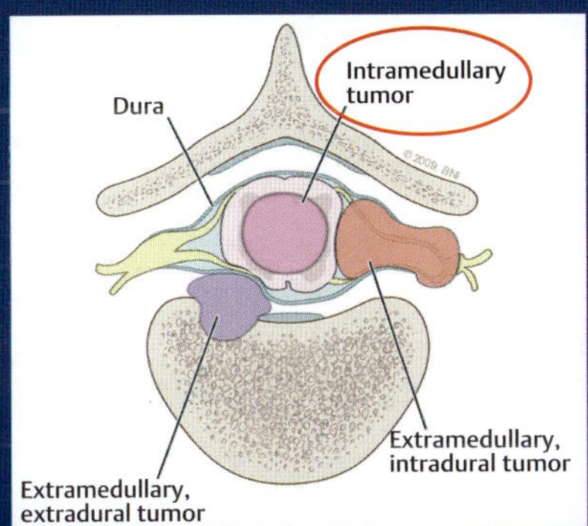

- Spinal tumors are classified as extradural, intradural extramedullary, or intradural intramedullary. Intradural intramedullary tumors are typically benign and originate within the spinal cord, causing invasion and destruction of both gray and white matter
- Symptoms include localized back or neck pain, radicular pain, sensory and motor deficits, bladder and bowel dysfunction, and gait disturbances

RADIOGRAPHIC FEATURES

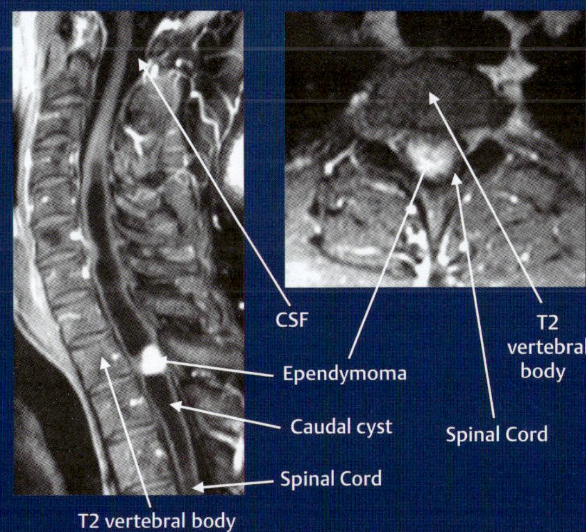

T1 MRI of a cervicothoracic intramedullary ependymoma with large rostral and caudal cysts

TREATMENT

- Intradural intramedullary tumors include benign tumors (epidermoid cysts and lipomas), glial tumors (ependymomas, astrocytomas, and gangliogliomas), and non-glial tumors (hemangioblastomas, lymphoma, and metastases)
- The goals of surgery include tissue diagnosis, tumor resection, and improvement of neurological function
- Adjuvant therapy, including radiotherapy and chemotherapy, is reserved for tumor recurrence, high-grade lesions, and contraindications to surgery

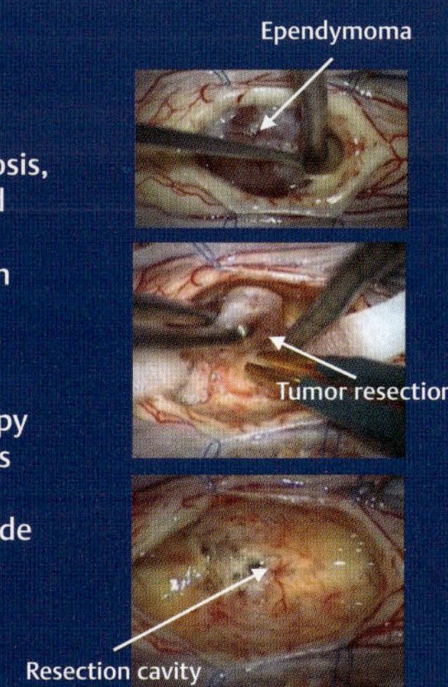

Further Reading

1. Das JM, Hoang S, Mesfin FB. Intramedullary Spinal Cord Tumors. In: StatPearls [Internet]. Treasure Island, FL: StatPearls Publishing; 2023

Nitin Agarwal
David T. Fernandes Cabral
Samuel Adida

Thieme

Lumbar Degenerative Disc Disease (DDD)

Lumbar degenerative disc disease without neurologic deficit is first managed conservatively with medications, physical therapy, and possibly epidural steroid injections

Red flag symptoms:
- Sudden loss of sensation in one or both legs, the groin and genital area, and/or the anal region
- "Cauda equina syndrome": Low back pain, pain that radiates down the leg, numbness around the anus, and loss of bowel or bladder control

Most common levels affected by lumbar DDD:
- L4-5
- L5-S1

ANATOMY

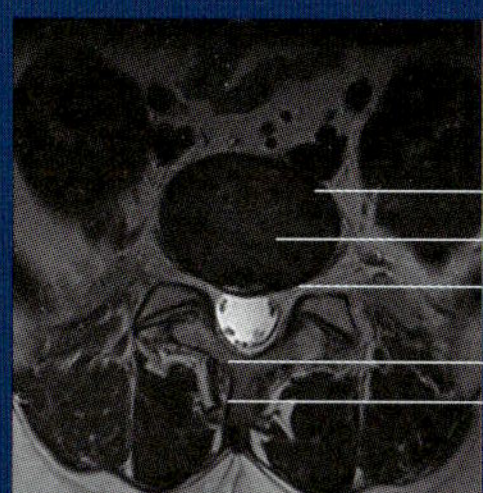

- Degenerative disc disease occurs when spinal discs degenerate or wear down
- The discs of the spine cushion the interlocking vertebrae and act as shock absorbers for the back, allowing it to bend, flex, and twist
- They break down over time as a natural part of the aging process
  - Dehydration of disc is part of pathology
- Lumbar DDD most commonly cause lumbar radiculopathy or "sciatica"
  - Pain, weakness, numbness, or tingling in the leg, buttocks, hips, or lower back.
  - Pain can be constant, sharp, or burning, and it can make it difficult to move the leg, foot, or toes

PATHOLOGY

Disc herniation

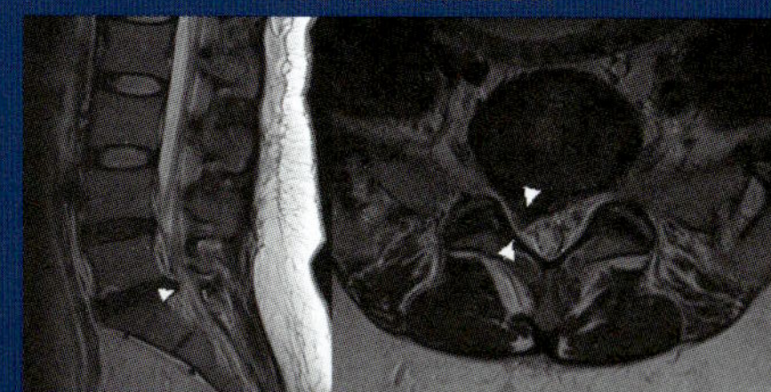

Spinal stenosis

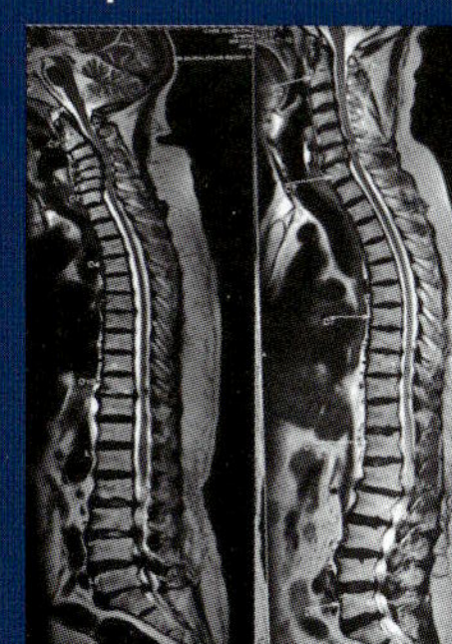

TREATMENT

- Conservative therapy:
  - Physical therapy
  - Pharmacological management (i.e., NSAID)
  - Epidural steroid injections
- Most patients experience relief from pain within a month or two with conservative treatment. When these treatments fail to provide relief, surgery may be indicated
- <u>SURGICAL INTERVENTION</u>
  - Discectomy
  - Laminectomy
  - Artificial disc replacement
  - Spinal Fusion

Further Reading

1. Saleem S, Aslam HM, Rehmani MA, Raees A, Alvi AA, Ashraf J. Lumbar disc degenerative disease: disc degeneration symptoms and magnetic resonance image findings. Asian Spine J 2013;7(4):322–334
2. Wang YX, Griffith JF, Zeng XJ et al. Prevalence and sex difference of lumbar disc space narrowing in elderly Chinese men and women: osteoporotic fractures in men (Hong Kong) and osteoporotic fractures in women (Hong Kong) studies. Arthritis Rheum 2013;65(4):1004–1010

Nitin Agarwal
David T. Fernandes Cabral
Regan Shanahan

Thieme

Lumbar Spine-Part I

Lumbar disk herniation is most common at L4–L5 and L5–S1 due to the high mechanical load and mobility

ANATOMY

- Vertebral bodies: The largest in the spine, especially in L4 and L5, to support body weight and shear forces
- The shape becomes more cylindrical with increasing size from L1 to L5
- Spinous processes: Short and broad in the lumbar region, providing attachment for muscles and ligaments
    - Less prominent than in the thoracic spine but can be palpated for tenderness or deformity
- Facet joints: Orientated sagittally in the lumbar spine, allowing flexion and extension while limiting rotation
    - Common site of degenerative changes, leading to facet joint osteoarthritis and stenosis
- Intervertebral disks: Disk heights increase and become more lordotic in the lower lumbar spine, contributing to increased motion and potential for degradation
- Spinal canal and nerve roots: The lumbar spinal canal is wide compared to the thoracic region, but stenosis can occur due to degenerative changes
- The cauda equina, a collection of lumbar, sacral, and coccygeal nerve roots, extends from L1 to L2 downward
- Conus medullaris: The tapered, lower end of the spinal cord; it is located at the level of the first or second lumbar vertebra (L1 or L2)

Biomechanics:

- The lumbar spine allows a high range of flexion and extension (forward bending and backward arching) but limited lateral bending and rotation
- The lumbosacral junction (L5–S1) is a critical weight-bearing area and commonly the site of pathology

Nitin Agarwal
David T. Fernandes Cabral
Samuel Adida

Thieme

Lumbar Spine-Part II

Spinal stenosis in the lumbar region, primarily affecting the L4–L5 area, results in narrowing of the spinal canal and nerve root compression commonly presents with neurogenic claudication

PHYSICAL EXAMINATION

Neurological considerations:
- The lumbar spinal cord terminates at L1–L2; below this, the cauda equina nerves carry sensory and motor function to the lower extremities and pelvic organs
- Lumbosacral nerve roots:
    - L3–L4: Knee extension (quadriceps), patellar reflex
    - L4–L5: Dorsiflexion (extensor hallucis longus), decreased sensation in the dorsum of the foot
    - L5–S1: Plantarflexion (gastrocnemius/soleus), Achilles reflex

1. Inspection: Assess for postural abnormalities like lordosis, scoliosis, or kyphosis; look for muscle atrophy or asymmetry, often indicative of nerve root impingement
2. Palpation: Palpate the spinous processes of L1–L5 for tenderness, step-offs (fractures), or deformities; palpate the paraspinal muscles to assess for spasm or tightness
    - Tenderness over sacroiliac joints may indicate referred pain from lumbar pathology
3. Range of motion (ROM): Flexion/extension, lateral flexion, rotation
4. Neurological testing:
    - Motor function: Test strength in major muscle groups (e.g., quadriceps, hamstrings, calf muscles)
    - Sensory function: Check for sensory loss along the L2–S1 dermatomes
    - Reflexes: Evaluate the patellar (L3–L4) and Achilles (S1) reflexes
    - Straight leg raise (SLR) test: Positive if pain radiates down the leg (indicative of lumbar nerve root compression, often due to disk herniation)
5. Special tests:
    - Crossed straight leg raise test: Pain in the opposite leg suggests a herniated disk
    - Valsalva maneuver: Increases intra-abdominal pressure and may reproduce radicular pain, indicating disk herniation

Nitin Agarwal
David T. Fernandes Cabral
Samuel Adida

Thieme

Lumbar Spine-Part III

Spondylolisthesis frequently occurs at L5–S1 caused by a defect in the pars interarticularis (spondylolysis)

PATHOLOGY & MANAGEMENT

Pathology:

- Herniated disk: Most commonly at L4–L5 and L5–S1, herniation can cause radiculopathy, often presenting with sharp, shooting pain in the leg, weakness, and sensory changes (commonly known as sciatica)
    - Sciatica is a common presentation due to compression of the sciatic nerve
- Lumbar spinal stenosis: Degenerative narrowing of the spinal canal, leading to neurogenic claudication (pain, numbness, and weakness in the legs with walking or standing)
    - Often associated with facet arthropathy and disk degeneration
- Spondylolisthesis: Forward displacement of one vertebra over another, typically at L5–S1, due to a defect or fracture of the pars interarticularis (spondylolysis)
    - Can cause back pain and nerve root compression
- Degenerative disk disease: Loss of disk height, dehydration, and disk bulging or herniation, leading to radicular pain or spinal stenosis
- Compression fractures: Often due to osteoporosis, trauma, or metastatic disease, usually affecting the vertebral bodies of the lumbar spine
- Cauda equina syndrome: A medical emergency resulting from compression of the cauda equina, causing saddle anesthesia, bowel and bladder dysfunction, and lower extremity weakness

Lumbar diskectomy:

- Indications: Symptomatic herniated disks causing radiculopathy or spinal cord compression
- Procedure: Removal of the herniated portion of the disk through a minimally invasive or open approach

Laminectomy and fusion:

- Indications: Spinal stenosis, degenerative disk disease, or spondylolisthesis
- Procedure: Decompression of the spinal canal with removal of the lamina, often followed by fusion using hardware to stabilize the spine

Posterior lumbar interbody fusion (PLIF):

- Indications: Instability, degenerative disk disease, or deformities like spondylolisthesis
- Procedure: Involves the removal of the disk and placement of a graft or cage between the vertebrae to promote fusion

Minimally invasive spine surgery (MISS):

- Indications: Herniated disks, stenosis, and spondylolisthesis
- Procedure: Utilizes smaller incisions and specialized instruments to perform decompression and fusion with less muscle dissection and faster recovery

Nitin Agarwal
David T. Fernandes Cabral
Samuel Adida

Thieme

Odontoid Pannus-Part I

Odontoid pannus is a soft tissue mass that forms at the atlantoaxial joint and can lead to spinal cord and vertebral artery compression

ETIOLOGY

- Odontoid pannus refers to the abnormal soft tissue mass or thickening that develops around the odontoid process (dens) of the C2 vertebra (the axis), specifically at the atlantoaxial joint

Etiology
- Rheumatoid arthritis is the most common cause of odontoid pannus. In RA, chronic synovitis (inflammation of the synovial lining) at the atlantoaxial joint leads to the development of a fibrous pannus that can impinge upon the odontoid process and cause spinal cord compression
    - The pannus is fibrotic, and it can lead to destruction of the cartilage and ligaments around the cervical spine, resulting in atlantoaxial instability
- Trauma:
    - C1–C2 dislocations or fractures can lead to fibrosis and the formation of a pannus around the odontoid process, especially if there is disruption of the ligamentous structures that support the atlantoaxial joint
- Other systemic diseases:
    - Ankylosing spondylitis, psoriatic arthritis, and reactive arthritis can also cause inflammation at the atlantoaxial joint, resulting in the formation of pannus
    - Systemic lupus erythematosus (SLE) or other autoimmune diseases may also lead to the development of an odontoid pannus

Further Reading

1. Greenberg MS. Greenberg's Handbook of Neurosurgery. 10th ed. New York, NY: Thieme Medical Publishing Group; 2023

Nitin Agarwal
David T. Fernandes Cabral
Regan Shanahan

Thieme

Odontoid Pannus-Part II

Imaging with MRI is the gold standard for diagnosing odontoid pannus and assessing its effect on the spinal cord and vertebral arteries. CT and X-rays are helpful for evaluating bone involvement and instability

PATHOPHYSIOLOGY

- The odontoid pannus is composed of granulation tissue, which is an inflammatory or fibrotic tissue that develops in response to prolonged inflammation. In the context of rheumatoid arthritis, this tissue is rich in inflammatory cells, including lymphocytes, plasma cells, and macrophages
- As the pannus grows, it can encroach upon the odontoid process, potentially causing compression of surrounding structures:
    - Spinal cord: Can lead to myelopathy with symptoms ranging from weakness, sensory loss, and gait disturbances to bladder/bowel dysfunction
    - Vertebral arteries: Compression of the vertebral arteries by the pannus can lead to vertebrobasilar insufficiency with symptoms such as dizziness, nausea, visual disturbances, and in severe cases, brainstem ischemia
- Nerve roots: Pannus may also compress the nerve roots exiting the cervical spine, leading to radiculopathy with pain, numbness, or weakness in the upper extremities

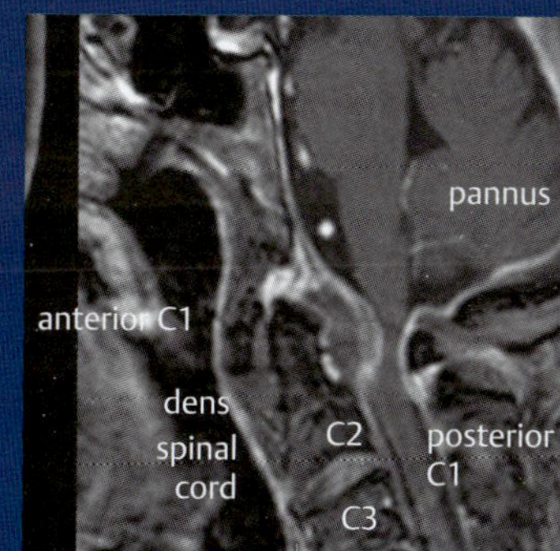

Nitin Agarwal
David T. Fernandes Cabral
Regan Shanahan

Thieme

Odontoid Pannus-Part III

Treatment may be conservative (e.g., DMARDs for RA) or surgical (e.g., odontoidectomy or posterior fusion) depending on the severity of neurological symptoms and spinal instability. Early intervention is critical to prevent permanent neurological damage

DIAGNOSIS & MANAGEMENT

Diagnosis
- X-rays: Lateral radiographs of the cervical spine may reveal an enlarged soft tissue mass in front of the odontoid process. Atlantoaxial subluxation may be visible
- CT scan: Provides better visualization of bone structures and can identify joint space narrowing, osteophytes, or fractures. It can also detect odontoid fractures or dislocations contributing to pannus formation
- MRI: MRI will show the pannus and can assess its size, location, and impact on the spinal cord. MRI can also evaluate the vertebral arteries for signs of compression
- Laboratory studies (when inflammatory diseases are suspected):
- Rheumatoid factor (RF) and anti-CCP antibodies: To assess for rheumatoid arthritis
- Erythrocyte sedimentation rate (ESR) and C-reactive protein (CRP): To evaluate the degree of inflammation
- Complete blood count (CBC) and serum uric acid may help in ruling out other potential causes such as gout or infection

Treatment

Medical Management
- Disease-modifying antirheumatic drugs (DMARDs) such as methotrexate or biologic agents (e.g., TNF inhibitors, rituximab) are used to control the underlying inflammatory process and limit pannus formation
- Nonsteroidal anti-inflammatory drugs (NSAIDs) can be used for symptomatic relief
- Corticosteroids can be used in flare-ups of rheumatoid arthritis but should be used with caution due to the risk of osteoporosis and spinal instability

Surgical Management:
- Odontoidectomy: This involves removing the odontoid process to relieve compression on the spinal cord
- Posterior cervical fusion (e.g., C1–C2 fusion): If there is atlantoaxial instability, posterior fusion with instrumentation (e.g., screws and rods) may be performed to restore stability
- Occipitocervical fusion: In cases of severe instability or deformity due to chronic rheumatoid arthritis, a fusion from the occiput to the cervical spine may be necessary

Nitin Agarwal
David T. Fernandes Cabral
Regan Shanahan

Thieme

Ossifying Fibromas

<1%

of all spinal tumors

Histological examination is necessary for diagnosis, as ossifying fibromas must be differentiated from:

- **Aneurysmal bone cysts**
- **Giant cell tumors**
- **Osteoid osteomas**
- **Osteoblastomas**

ETIOLOGY

- Ossifying fibromas are benign tumors characterized by the replacement of normal bone with a fibrous cellular stroma
- They most commonly occur in the mandible and maxilla. Ossifying fibromas of the spine are rare

PRESENTATION

- Signs and symptoms of spinal cord or nerve root compression:
    - Localized back or neck pain
    - Radicular pain
    - Sensory and motor deficits
    - Bladder and bowel dysfunction
    - Gait disturbances

HISTOLOGIC FEATURES

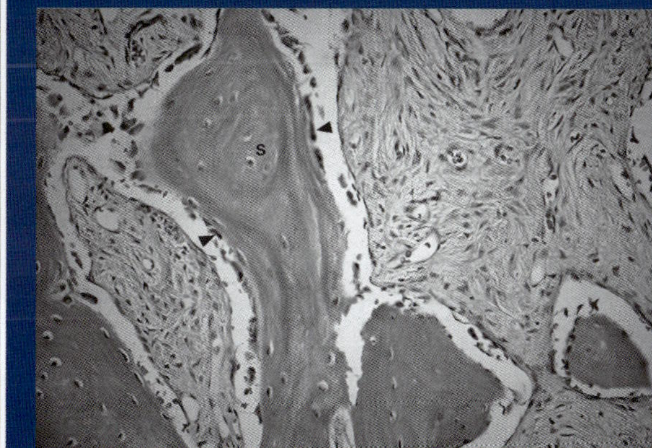

Ossifying fibromas are characterized by the presence of mature lamellar bony spicules (S), rimmed by osteoblasts (arrowheads), and mixed with fibrous stroma

TREATMENT

- Ossifying fibromas are slow-growing tumors that are initially asymptomatic until they invade the local surrounding structures
- High recurrence rates, ranging from 30 to 58%, have been reported after curettage and enucleation
- Recurrence after complete resection is rare. However, as ossifying fibromas have the potential for malignant transformation, total surgical excision is preferred when possible

Further Reading

1. Yang J et al. Ossifying fibroma of the cervical spine: first case report and literature review. World Neurosurg 2020;140:247–250

Nitin Agarwal
David T. Fernandes Cabral
Samuel Adida

Thieme

Osteoblastomas

1%

of all spinal tumors

Key differences between osteoid osteomas and osteoblastoma:

- **Osteoid osteomas are smaller, lack growth potential, and commonly occur in long bones (e.g., femur, tibia), whereas osteoblastomas are larger, more vascular, and are more frequently found in the axial skeleton**
- **Osteoid osteomas cause night pain relieved by NSAIDs, whereas osteoblastoma pain is less likely to worsen at night and is less responsive to NSAIDs**
- **Osteoid osteomas can often be managed non-surgically or with minimally invasive procedures, whereas osteoblastomas require surgical resection and have a higher recurrence rate**

PRESENTATION

- Osteoblastoma is a benign bone-forming tumor characterized by the production of osteoid and immature bone trabeculae. This tumor has a strong predilection for the spine and can locally recur, with a rare potential for malignant transformation into osteosarcoma
- Osteoblastoma generally presents as a well-demarcated, mixed lytic and sclerotic lesion on imaging
- Clinical manifestations often arise from spinal cord or nerve root compression and may include localized back or neck pain, radicular pain, sensory or motor deficits, bladder and bowel dysfunction, and gait disturbances

RADIOGRAPHIC FEATURES

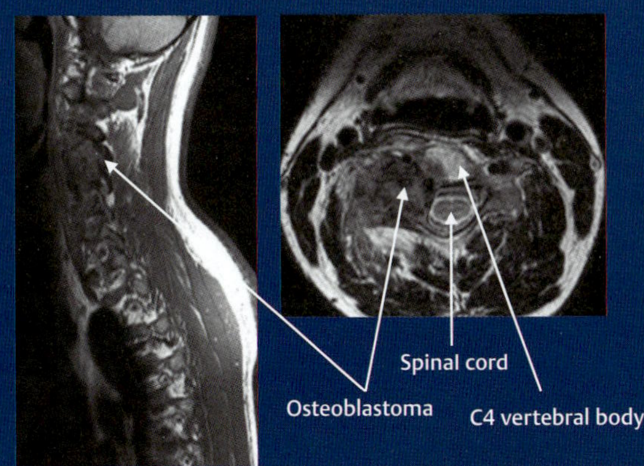

T1 and T2 MRI of a cervical osteoblastoma with epidural involvement

TREATMENT

- Osteoid osteoma and osteoblastoma are histologically indistinguishable but are differentiated by size and clinical behavior. Osteoid osteomas are smaller and typically responsive to NSAIDs, while osteoblastomas are larger, more aggressive, and often cause pain that does not respond to NSAIDs. Osteoblastomas are also more aggressive both clinically and radiographically compared to osteoid osteomas
- Osteoblastomas are relatively resistant to traditional radiotherapy and chemotherapy, making surgical intervention the primary treatment
- Complete excision offers pain relief in 93% of patients, though the recurrence rate is approximately 10%. Early diagnosis and thorough surgical removal are critical for effective management

Further Reading

1. Wu M, Xu K, Xie Y et al. Diagnostic and management options of osteoblastoma in the spine. Med Sci Monit 2019;25:1362–1372
2. Greenberg MS. Greenberg's Handbook of Neurosurgery. 10th ed. Stuttgart, Germany: Thieme Medical Publishing Group; 2023

Nitin Agarwal
David T. Fernandes Cabral
Samuel Adida

Thieme

Osteochondromas

4%
of all spinal tumors

Imaging characteristics:
- CT shows medullary continuity and the cartilage cap more clearly than radiographs. Septal enhancement between cartilage lobules may also be seen
- MRI can evaluate cartilage thickness, which is associated with malignant potential. Benign lesions enhance peripherally with contrast, while chondrosarcoma may show septal enhancement

PRESENTATION

- Osteochondroma is the most common benign bone tumor, accounting for 36% of benign bone tumors. While typically found in long bones, spinal osteochondromas are relatively rare, representing 4–7% of primary benign spinal tumors and less than 3% of all osteochondromas
- They may occur as solitary lesions or as part of multiple hereditary exostoses, an inherited autosomal dominant condition
- Osteochondroma has a low risk of malignant transformation, with an estimated risk of 1% for solitary lesions and up to 3% to 5% when associated with multiple hereditary exostosis. Solitary lesions are more frequent than those associated with multiple hereditary exostosis
- Spinal osteochondromas may present with symptoms such as localized back or neck pain, radicular pain, sensory and motor deficits, bladder and bowel dysfunction, and gait disturbances

RADIOGRAPHIC FEATURES

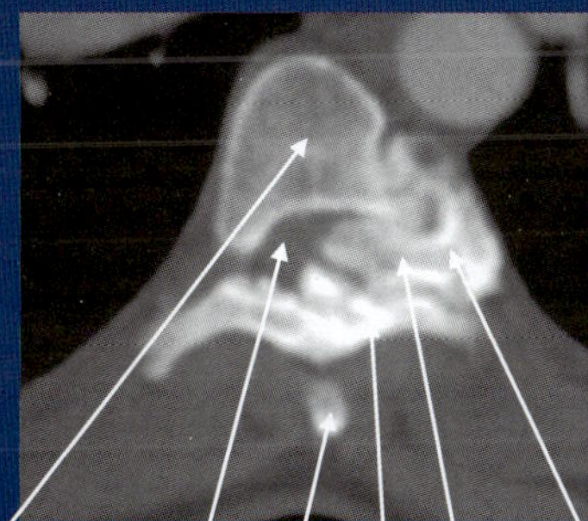

An osteochondroma involving the left pedicle of a thoracic vertebra extending into the spinal cord, displacing the thecal sac and spinal cord

TREATMENT

- The cervical spine is the most frequently affected site, although lesions causing spinal cord compression are relatively rare
- Treatment for spinal osteochondromas begins with a thorough history and exam to assess genetic inheritance and rule out neurovascular compromise, which may require surgery. Most lesions are benign, painless, and managed with observation and radiographic surveillance
- Intractable pain, radiculopathy, myelopathy, or vascular compression warrant surgical intervention, which may involve marginal or wide excision using posterior, anterior, or combined approaches, with or without stabilization or fusion. Complete resection of the cartilage cap is crucial to minimize recurrence risk, especially in pediatric patients
- Recurrence rates reported in the literature range from 0 to 4%

Further Reading

1. Lotfinia I, Vahedi A, Aeinfar K et al. Cervical osteochondroma with neurological symptoms: literature review and a case report. Spinal Cord Ser Cases 2017;3:16038
2. Rajakulasingam R, Murphy J, Botchu R et al. Osteochondromas of the cervical spine-case series and review. J Clin Orthop Trauma 2020;11(5):905–909
3. Yakkanti R, Onyekwelu I, Carreon LY et al. Solitary osteochondroma of the spine-a case series: review of solitary osteochondroma with myelopathic symptoms. Global Spine J 2018;8(4):323–339
4. Greenberg MS. Greenberg's Handbook of Neurosurgery. 10th ed. Stuttgart, Germany: Thieme Medical Publishing Group; 2023

Nitin Agarwal
David T. Fernandes Cabral
Samuel Adida

Thieme

Osteoid Osteomas (OO)

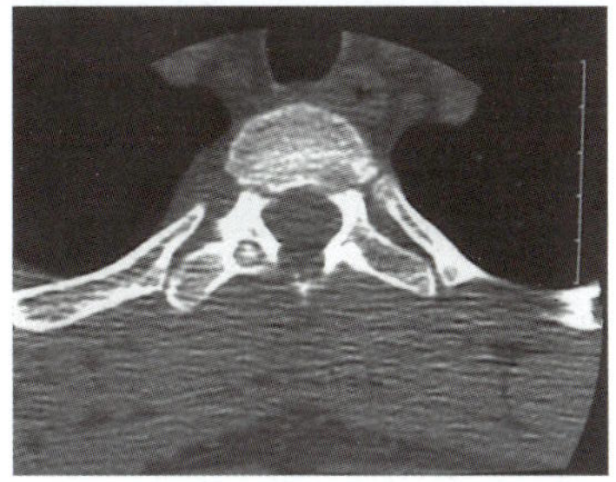

Histologically identical
- <2 cm = osteoid osteoma
- >2 cm osteoblastoma

Benign bone tumors have a high cure rate with complete excision

CLINICAL PRESENTATION

General
- Osteoid osteoma (OO) is a benign (noncancerous) bone tumor that typically forms in young adults
- Osteoblastoma (OB) is a rare, benign locally recurrent tumor with a predilection for the spine that may rarely undergo sarcomatous change to osteosarcoma
- OBs are more vascular than OOs
- OOs occur in long bones of skeleton

Signs and Symptoms
- Characteristically cause night pain and pain relieved by aspirin
- Tenderness confined to vicinity of the lesion occurs in 60%
- 28% patients with OB present with myelopathy
- 22% patients with OO present with neurological deficit

Differential Diagnosis
Lesions with similar symptoms and increased uptake on radionuclide bone scan
- Benign OB
- OO: More pronounced sclerosis of adjacent bone than benign OB
- Osteogenic sarcoma
- Aneurysmal bone cyst
- Unilateral pedicle/laminar necrosis

COMPARISON

Comparison of osteoid osteoma and benign osteoblastoma

	Osteoid osteoma	Benign osteoblastoma
Percent of primary bone tumors	3.2%	
Percent of primary vertebral tumors	1.4%	
Percent that occur in spine	10%	35%
Size limitations	≤ 1 cm	> 1 cm
Growth pattern	Confined, self limiting	More extensive, may extend into spinal canal
Potential for malignant change?	No	Rare
Location within spine (83 patients)		
▸ % in cervical spine	27%	25%
▸ % in thoracic spine		35%
▸ % in lumbar region	59%	35%
Location within vertebra (81 patients)		
▸ Lamina only	33%	16%
▸ Pedicle only	15%	32%
▸ Articular facet only	19%	0
▸ Vertebral body (VB) only	7%	5%
▸ Transverse process only	6%	8%
▸ Spinous process	5%	5%
▸ > 1 element of neural arch	6%	19%
▸ Combined posterior elements & VB	0	11%

Data from *Greenberg MS. Greenberg's handbook of neurosurgery. 10th ed. New york, NY: Thieme medical publishing group; 2023.

EVALUATION & TREATMENT

Evaluation
- Bone scans are sensitive to detect OO/BOB
- Caution regarding needle biopsy: If the lesion is osteosarcoma, there is risk of seeding in the contaminated needle tract
- OO: Radiolucent area with or without surrounding density, often isolated to pedicle or facet. May not show on tomograms
- OB: Most are expansile, destructive lesions, contralateral spondylosis
    - 17% having moderate sclerosis
    - 31% have areas of increased density 20% have calcified shell

Treatment
- Cure is dependent on complete excision
- OO: Cortical bone may be thickened, with granulomatous mass in underlying cavity
- OB: Hemorrhagic, friable, red, purple mass, well circumscribed
    - Complete excision is associated with pain resolution in 93% of patients
    - Recurrence rate with complete excision = 10%

Further Readings

1. Meyers SP, ed. Differential Diagnosis in Neuroimaging: Spine. Stuttgart: Thieme Medical Publishers; 2016
2. Mattle H, Mumenthaler M, Taub E, eds. Fundamentals of Neurology: An Illustrated Guide. 2nd ed. Stuttgart: Thieme Medical Publishers; 2016
3. Greenberg MS. Greenberg's Handbook of Neurosurgery. 10th ed. New York, NY: Thieme Medical Publishing Group; 2023

Nitin Agarwal
David T. Fernandes Cabral
Regan Shanahan

Thieme

Osteosarcomas

3–5%
of all spinal tumors

Genetic risk
Rb, p53,
Li-Fraumeni syndrome,* and *Bloom syndrome

Male > Female

PRESENTATION

- Osteosarcoma is the second most common primary bone tumor, yet spinal involvement is rare, occurring in only 3–5% of cases. At the molecular level, osteosarcoma exhibits significant genetic complexity, with several genetic disorders linked to its development
- Spinal osteosarcoma predominantly arises in the lumbosacral region, typically affecting males in their 40s, and may occasionally develop from preexisting conditions such as osteoblastoma or Paget's disease
- Pain is the hallmark symptom, reported by nearly all patients, while over 70% experience neurological deficits. Its clinical presentation may include:
  - Localized back or neck pain
  - Radicular pain
  - Sensory and motor deficits
  - Bladder and bowel dysfunction
  - Gait abnormalities

RADIOGRAPHIC FEATURES

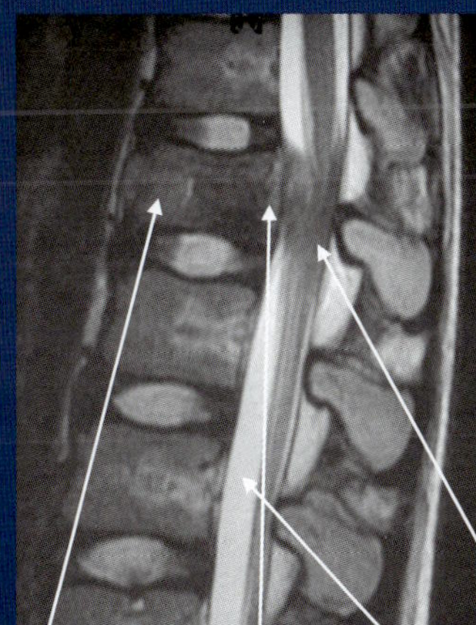

CT of osteosarcoma involving the L1 vertebra, associated with cortical destruction and epidural extension

TREATMENT

- Management of spinal osteosarcoma is challenging due to its complexity. Wide en bloc resection, when feasible, offers the best survival outcomes, especially with chemotherapy and radiation
- Tumor location often necessitates intralesional resection for critical structures like pedicles or the vertebral artery foramen. Preoperative planning is vital to address complications such as nerve root sacrifice, blood loss, and implant failure
- Non-surgical treatments, including radiation and chemotherapy, are essential for inoperable or residual disease. Despite advancements, spinal osteosarcoma has a five-year survival rate of 30–40%, significantly lower than extremity cases. Emerging therapies, such as carbon ion radiotherapy and novel chemotherapeutics, may improve outcomes

Further Reading
1. Katonis P, Datsis G, Karantanas A et al. Spinal osteosarcoma. Clin Med Insights Oncol 2013;7:199–208
2. Greenberg MS. Greenberg's Handbook of Neurosurgery. 10th ed. Stuttgart, Germany: Thieme Medical Publishing Group; 2023

Nitin Agarwal
David T. Fernandes Cabral
Samuel Adida

Thieme

Pediatric Spinal Tumors

The most common pediatric spinal tumors are intramedullary (astrocytoma)

The most common symptom of a spinal tumor in a child is chronic back or neck pain

50% of pediatric spinal tumors are in the cervico-thoracic region and usually affect a small number of vertebrae

PRESENTATION

- 25–30% of children with a spinal cord tumor suffer from recurrent episodes of back pain
- Symptoms include
  - Motor weakness in arms and legs
  - Progressive scoliosis
  - Gait disturbance
  - Muscle rigidity with paraspinal muscle spasm
  - Numbness or tingling in the arms and legs
  - Poor bladder or bowel control

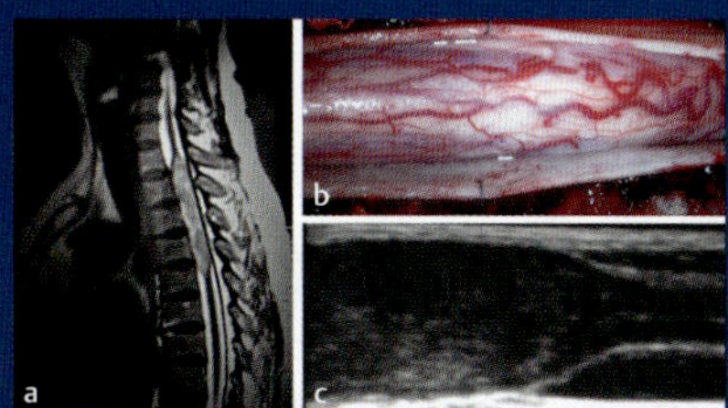

CLASSIFICATION

- Intramedullary tumors (gliomas [90–95%]: pilocytic and anaplastic astrocytomas [60%] and ependymomas [30%])

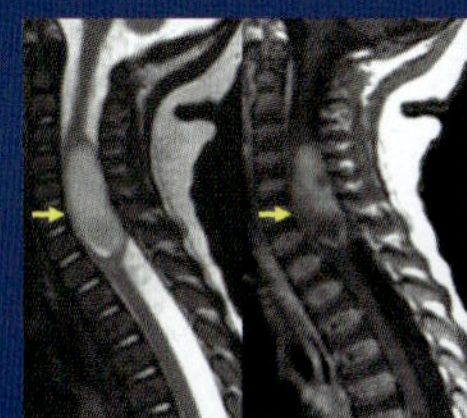

- Intradural, extramedullary tumors

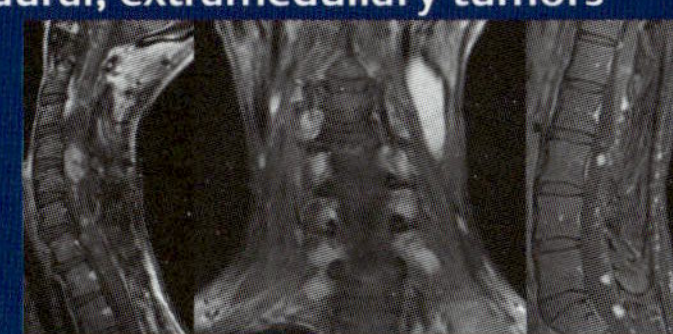

- Extradural tumors
  - Primary bone tumors
  - Metastatic tumors

OTHER CONSIDERATIONS

- Pediatric spine anatomy and physiology are dynamic and vary with age
- Children exhibit a higher frequency of congenital malformations and genetic syndromes
- Diagnosis is often delayed due to non-specific features and waxing and waning pain symptoms
- MRI is gold standard for diagnosis

INTERVENTION

- Spinal tumors are often treated with a multidisciplinary approach to alleviate spinal cord compression and prevent neurologic deficits
  - Intra-operative biopsy
  - Surgery (tumor debulking)
  - Radiation
  - Chemotherapy
  - Targeted immunotherapy drugs

Further Reading

1. Huisman TA. Pediatric tumors of the spine. Cancer Imag 2009;9(Special issue A):S45–S48
2. Ho ML. Pediatric spine tumors and dysontogenetic masses. Neuroimaging Clin N Am. 2023;33(3):375–388

Nitin Agarwal
David T. Fernandes Cabral
Samuel Adida

Thieme

Pott's Disease-Part I

Pott's disease presents with chronic back pain, progressive kyphosis, and late-onset neurological deficits, requiring a high index of suspicion in endemic regions and immunosuppressed patients

CLINICAL OVERVIEW

Introduction

- Pott's disease, or spinal tuberculosis (TB spondylodiskitis), is a chronic granulomatous infection of the spine caused by *Mycobacterium tuberculosis*. It is the most common form of skeletal TB (~50%), with a predilection for the thoracic spine and a high risk of progressive vertebral destruction, kyphotic deformity, and spinal cord compression. Delayed diagnosis increases morbidity due to its insidious presentation and high potential for neurological compromise

Pathophysiology

- Hematogenous dissemination from a primary pulmonary focus (often subclinical)
- Infection initially affects the anterior vertebral body, leading to progressive caseous necrosis, vertebral collapse, and kyphotic deformity ("gibbus deformity")
- Unlike pyogenic infections, TB spondylitis frequently spares the disk in early stages
- Paraspinal abscess formation ("cold abscess") is common, often extending into the psoas muscle without significant systemic inflammation

Clinical Presentation

- Gradual onset back pain (weeks to months), often without fever
- Neurological deficits (30–50%) due to spinal cord compression from vertebral collapse or epidural extension
- Kyphotic deformity ("gibbus") from progressive vertebral body destruction
- Systemic symptoms: Low-grade fever, night sweats, weight loss (variable)

Nitin Agarwal
David T. Fernandes Cabral
Regan Shanahan

Thieme

Pott's Disease-Part II

Medical management with prolonged anti-TB therapy (≥6–12 months) is the cornerstone of treatment, with surgery reserved for neurological compromise, severe kyphosis, or instability

Key risk factors include endemic exposure, HIV/AIDS, immunosuppression, malnutrition, and untreated pulmonary TB, necessitating early screening in high-risk populations

DIAGNOSIS

- MRI with contrast (gold standard):
    - Hypointense T1, hyperintense T2 lesions with vertebral body destruction and prevertebral abscess formation
- Relative disk preservation in early disease (differentiates from pyogenic osteomyelitis)
- Rim-enhancing paraspinal or epidural abscess without significant inflammatory edema
- CT-guided biopsy: Essential for definitive diagnosis (caseating granulomas, AFB stain, GeneXpert MTB/RIF)
- Lab markers:↑ ESR/CRP (nonspecific)
- Tuberculin skin test (PPD) and IGRA (QuantiFERON-TB) may be positive but do not confirm active disease

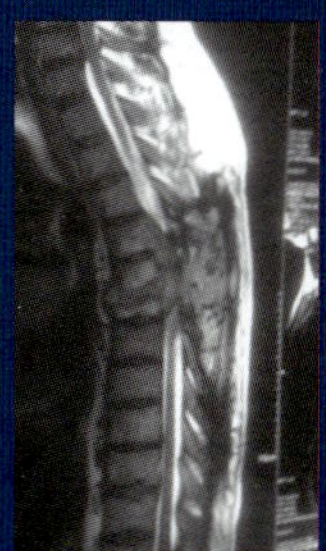

Preoperative magnetic resonance imaging (MRI) of dorsal spine shows Pott's disease involving T6–T7 vertebrae

MANAGEMENT

- First-line: Anti-TB therapy (6–12 months minimum):
    - RIPE regimen: Rifampin, isoniazid, pyrazinamide, ethambutol for 2 months, then rifampin + isoniazid for 4–10 months
    - Extended duration (12–18 months) if severe disease or poor response
- Surgical indications (reserved for select cases):
    - Neurological deficits (cord compression from abscess or deformity)
    - Severe kyphosis (>30–40 degrees) or progressive instability
    - Failure of medical therapy (persistent infection, worsening pain, or deformity)
- Procedures: Anterior corpectomy with reconstruction ± posterior stabilization

Nitin Agarwal
David T. Fernandes Cabral
Regan Shanahan

Thieme

Sacral Spine-Part I

Cauda equina syndrome, often caused by disk herniation, tumors, or trauma, results in compression of the sacral nerve roots. Symptoms include saddle anesthesia, bladder/bowel dysfunction, and lower extremity weakness

ANATOMY

Sacrum: Composed of five fused vertebrae (S1–S5) that form a wedge-shaped structure
- The sacral promontory is a key bony landmark at the anterior aspect of the sacrum, useful for pelvic imaging
- Sacral foramina (anterior and posterior) allow for the passage of sacral nerve roots, which are part of the cauda equina

Coccyx: Composed of 3–5 fused rudimentary vertebrae, the coccyx provides attachment for muscles and ligaments
- It is important for pelvic floor stability and is clinically relevant in cases of trauma or pain (coccydynia)

Sacrococcygeal joint: The junction between the sacrum and coccyx, which may become a source of pain or dysfunction, especially after trauma

Function and biomechanics:
- The sacrum transmits the body's weight from the spine to the pelvis and lower limbs, playing a vital role in posture and ambulation
- The sacroiliac joints, where the sacrum articulates with the ilium, are crucial for stability and force distribution between the upper body and the lower extremities

Nitin Agarwal
David T. Fernandes Cabral
Samuel Adida

Thieme

Sacral Spine-Part II

Sacral fracture fixation, typically involving screws and rods, is performed to stabilize the fracture and prevent further neurological compromise

PHYSICAL EXAMINATION

Neurological considerations:
- The sacral nerves are part of the cauda equina that innervates the lower extremities and pelvic organs (bladder, bowel, and sexual function)
- The S1–S5 nerve roots exit the sacrum through the sacral foramina and innervate the lower limbs and pelvic floor

1. Inspection: Inspect for deformities or asymmetry, especially in the sacrum and coccyx, which may indicate trauma, congenital defects, or degenerative changes
   - Look for signs of swelling, redness, or bruising at the sacral or coccygeal level, which may be indicative of trauma (e.g., coccygodynia or fractures)
2. Palpation: Palpate the sacrum for tenderness, especially over the sacroiliac joint, which can be painful in conditions like sacroiliitis or sacroiliac joint dysfunction; palpate the coccyx for tenderness or signs of coccydynia, which may arise from trauma or prolonged sitting
3. Range of motion (ROM):
   - Pelvic tilt test: Assess for any pain or abnormal motion in the pelvis, which may indicate sacroiliac joint dysfunction
   - Limited or painful movement during flexion, extension, or lateral tilting of the pelvis can be indicative of issues in the sacral region or the sacroiliac joints
4. Neurological testing:
   - Saddle anesthesia: Assess for sensory changes in the perineum and buttocks, which may indicate cauda equina syndrome
   - Check for any signs of bladder, bowel, or sexual dysfunction, which may be associated with sacral nerve involvement or cauda equina syndrome
5. Special tests:
   - Faber's/Patrick's test (figure-4 test): Assess for sacroiliac joint dysfunction or pelvic pathology by placing the patient in a figure-4 position and applying downward pressure
   - Straight leg raise test: Positive for pain radiating down the leg may indicate compression of sacral nerve roots or radiculopathy

Nitin Agarwal
David T. Fernandes Cabral
Samuel Adida

Thieme

Sacral Spine-Part III

Dysfunction of the sacroiliac joint, often due to degeneration, inflammation (e.g., ankylosing spondylitis), or trauma, can cause significant low back and buttock pain

PATHOLOGY & MANAGEMENT

Pathology:
- Sacral fractures: Sacral fractures typically occur due to trauma (e.g., falls, motor vehicle accidents) or as a result of osteoporosis
    - Symptoms include localized pain and potential neurological deficits if the fracture involves the sacral canal or nerve roots
- Cauda equina syndrome: A neurological emergency involving compression of the cauda equina, often resulting from disk herniation, tumors, or trauma
- Symptoms include saddle anesthesia, bladder/bowel dysfunction, and lower extremity weakness
- Sacroiliitis: Inflammation of the sacroiliac joints, often seen in inflammatory conditions like ankylosing spondylitis
    - Presents with low back pain, buttock pain, and stiffness, especially with activity
- Coccydynia: Pain localized to the coccyx, often resulting from trauma (e.g., falls onto the tailbone) or prolonged sitting
    - It can cause significant discomfort and may require conservative management or injections
- Congenital anomalies: Sacralization of the lumbar spine (where L5 fuses with the sacrum) or lumbarization of the sacrum (where S1 behaves like a lumbar vertebra) can lead to altered biomechanics and back pain
    - Spina bifida occulta may also be identified at the sacral level in some patients

Sacral fracture fixation:
- Indications: Significant fractures that compromise the spinal canal, nerve roots, or pelvic stability
- Procedure: Surgical stabilization using screws, rods, or plates, often in conjunction with other spinal fixation techniques

Sacroiliac joint fusion:
- Indications: Chronic pain from sacroiliac joint dysfunction that does not respond to conservative treatments
- Procedure: Fusion of the sacroiliac joint using screws or a minimally invasive approach, offering stability and pain relief

Cauda equina decompression surgery:
- Indications: Acute compression of the cauda equina due to herniated disks, tumors, or trauma
- Procedure: *Laminectomy*, decompression of the neural elements by removing the offending disk, bone, or tumor to relieve pressure on the cauda equina

Coccygectomy:
- Indications: Severe, persistent coccydynia that does not respond to conservative treatments (e.g., corticosteroid injections)
- Procedure: Surgical excision of the coccyx to alleviate pain

Nitin Agarwal
David T. Fernandes Cabral
Samuel Adida

Thieme

Spinal Angiosarcomas

<1%
of all spinal tumors

Genetic risk
NF1, *NF2*,
BRCA 1, and *BRCA 2*

- Complete surgical resection is ideal but often limited by the involvement of critical structures
- Preoperative embolization may reduce intraoperative bleeding
- Subtotal resection is associated with a high recurrence rate, and chemotherapy and radiation may be used as adjuvant therapies

ETIOLOGY

- Angiosarcomas are rare malignant vascular tumors that comprise 2% of all sarcomas
- Primary angiosarcomas account for 1% of all angiosarcomas, and angiosarcoma of the spine is extremely rare

PRESENTATION

- Signs and symptoms of spinal cord or nerve root compression:
  - Localized back or neck pain
  - Radicular pain
  - Sensory and motor deficits
  - Bladder and bowel dysfunction
  - Gait disturbances

RADIOGRAPHIC FEATURES

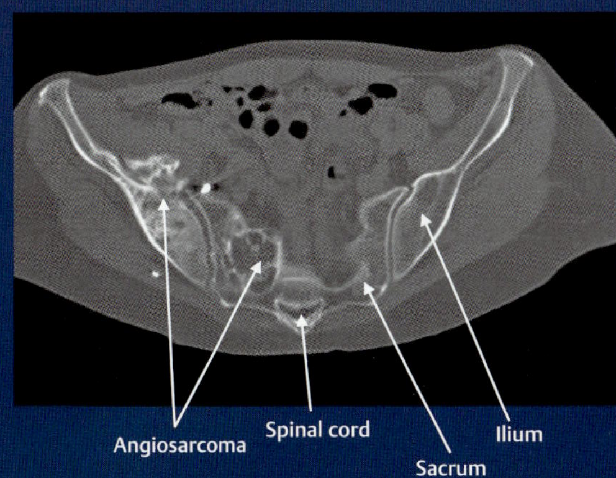

CT of irregular osteolytic lesions due to metastatic angiosarcoma. Lesions are observed in the right ilium and right sacral spine

OTHER CONSIDERATIONS

- Features of angiosarcomas include osteolytic lesions, ill-defined margins, and erosion of the cortex with soft-tissue involvement

TREATMENT

- Complete surgical resection with negative margins is the mainstay of treatment; however, this is not always possible due to involvement or invasion of surrounding structures such as spinal cord, dura, lungs, or major blood vessels
- Angiosarcomas are inherently vascular tumors with high potential for intraoperative bleeding. Preoperative endovascular embolization can be considered
- Subtotal resection has a high incidence of local recurrence. Chemotherapy and radiation therapy can be used as adjuvant therapies

Further Reading

1. Pülhorn H, Elliot T, Clark J, Gonzalvo A. Case report: angiosarcoma of the cervical spine. J Clin Neurosci 2017;45:129–131
2. Nacar OA, Ulu MO, Pekmezci M, Deviren V, Christopher AMES. Successful treatment of a very rare angiosarcoma involving the lumbar spine via en-bloc resection and radiotherapy: case report. Turk Neurosurg 2014;24(1):140–145

Nitin Agarwal
David T. Fernandes Cabral
Samuel Adida

Thieme

Spinal Deformity Measurements-Part I

CVA assesses cervical spine lordosis, with deviations linked to neck pain and postural issues

LL is essential in evaluating lumbar spine alignment, guiding treatment for lumbar degenerative diseases and deformities

CERVICAL/GLOBAL

Cervical vertebral angle (CVA):

- Definition: The CVA measures the alignment of the cervical spine in the sagittal plane
- Measurement:
    - Draw a line along the inferior endplate of C2 (the second cervical vertebra) and another line along the superior endplate of C7 (the seventh cervical vertebra)
    - Measure the angle formed between these two lines. This is the CVA
- Clinical relevance: A decrease in CVA can indicate cervical kyphosis, which may require surgical intervention

Sagittal vertical axis (SVA):

- Definition: The SVA measures the horizontal displacement of the C7 vertebral body relative to the posterior sacral promontory
- Measurement:
    - Drop a vertical plumb line from the center of C7 (the seventh cervical vertebra)
    - Measure the horizontal distance from this line to the sacral promontory (the front of the sacrum at the level of S1)
    - The horizontal distance from the plumb line to the sacral promontory is the SVA
- Clinical relevance: SVA >5 cm indicates global sagittal imbalance, often requiring surgical intervention to restore spinal alignment and improve function
    - Normal physiologic SVA will increase with age

THORACIC

Thoracic kyphosis (TK):

- Definition: TK is the angle of curvature of the thoracic spine in the sagittal plane, important for assessing kyphotic deformities
- Measurement:
    - Draw a line along the superior endplate of T4 and another line along the inferior endplate of T12
- Clinical relevance: An increase in TK can lead to postural deformities and pulmonary complications

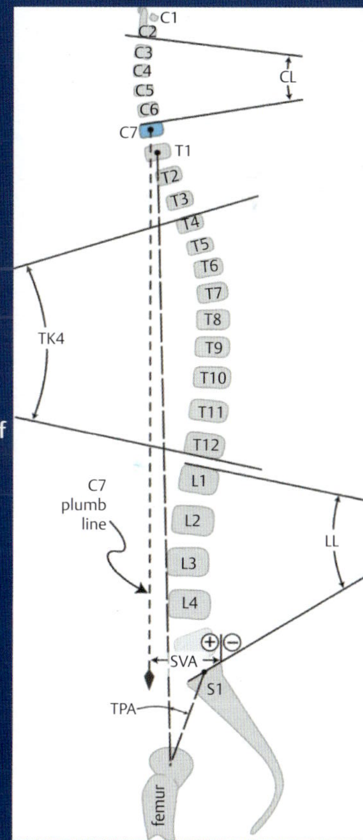

Nitin Agarwal
David T. Fernandes Cabral
Samuel Adida

Thieme

Spinal Deformity Measurements-Part II

PI is a fixed anatomical measurement that correlates with lumbar lordosis and influences sagittal spinal balance, affecting surgical planning for spinal deformities

LUMBAR

Lumbar lordosis (LL):
- Definition: LL measures the curvature of the lumbar spine in the sagittal plane, important for evaluating lumbar spine alignment and posture
- Measurement:
    - Identify the superior endplate of L1 and the inferior endplate of L5
    - Draw a line along the superior endplate of L1 and another line along the superior endplate of S1
- Clinical relevance: Decreased LL can indicate flat back deformity, while excessive lordosis can indicate lumbar instability

Sacral slope (SS):
- Definition: SS measures the angle between the horizontal line and the superior endplate of S1 (the first sacral vertebra)
- Measurement:
    - Draw a horizontal line at the top of the S1 endplate
    - Draw a line along the superior endplate of S1
- Clinical relevance: A low SS may be associated with flat back deformity or hypolordosis

Pelvic incidence (PI):
- Definition: PI is a fixed anatomical angle reflecting pelvic orientation relative to the lumbar spine
- Measurement:
    - Identify the center of the femoral head and the midpoint of the sacral endplate at S1
    - Draw a line from the femoral head center to the midpoint of the S1 endplate and a line perpendicular to the superior endplate of S1
- Clinical relevance: PI is a fixed measure and can influence the LL and pelvic tilt. It is used to assess pelvic orientation and spinal balance

Nitin Agarwal
David T. Fernandes Cabral
Samuel Adida

Thieme

Spinal Dural Arteriovenous Fistula-Part I

Spinal dural arteriovenous fistulas (SDAVFs) primarily affect middle-aged to older adults (typically 40–70 years old), with a slight male predominance

CLINICAL OVERVIEW

Introduction

- SDAVFs are abnormal connections between dural arteries and the epidural venous plexus, leading to increased venous pressure and spinal cord ischemia. They are the most common cause of acquired spinal vascular malformations and typically present with progressive myelopathy due to venous congestion and secondary spinal cord ischemia. SDAVFs are most commonly located in the thoracolumbar region (T12–L2) but can occur anywhere along the spinal cord

Pathophysiology and Classification

- Mechanism: SDAVFs result from abnormal arteriovenous shunting where radicular arteries (typically from the segmental spinal arteries) feed into the dural venous plexus. This leads to elevated venous pressure in the epidural veins, which then drains into the spinal cord parenchyma, causing ischemia and edema
- Venous congestion leads to dorsal spinal cord ischemia, which typically manifests as motor weakness, sensory deficits, and bladder dysfunction
- Classification:
    - Type I (classic SDAVF): Direct connection between radicular arteries and the venous plexus. Most common
    - Type II (perimedullary AVF): Arterial supply from larger vessels that supply the spinal cord and vein, causing severe cord compression

Nitin Agarwal
David T. Fernandes Cabral
Regan Shanahan

Thieme

Spinal Dural Arteriovenous Fistula-Part II

MRI with contrast is the first-line imaging modality for identifying SDAVF, but digital subtraction angiography (DSA) is the gold standard for definitive diagnosis and treatment planning

PRESENTATION & DIAGNOSIS

Presentation
- Progressive myelopathy with motor weakness (especially lower extremities)
- Sensory deficits: Numbness, paresthesias, or loss of proprioception, most often below the level of the fistula
- Bladder and bowel dysfunction: Difficulty with urination or defecation, indicative of cauda equina involvement or spinal cord compression
- Exacerbation with activity: Symptoms may worsen with standing, walking, or straining due to increased venous pressure
- Onset: Symptoms typically evolve over months to years, but early detection is critical to prevent permanent neurological damage

Imaging
- MRI of the spine (gold standard)
- Contrast-enhanced MRI is critical for identifying venous congestion and spinal cord edema (dorsal column involvement)
    - Look for “flow voids” on T2-weighted images in the epidural venous plexus, indicating abnormal vascularity
    - Spinal cord swelling and hyperintensity may also be seen
- DSA: Gold standard for definitive diagnosis and localization of the fistula
    - DSA helps visualize the feeding artery, shunt, and draining veins, which is crucial for treatment planning (endovascular embolization)
- CT angiography: Occasionally used for an initial assessment or in the cases where DSA is not available

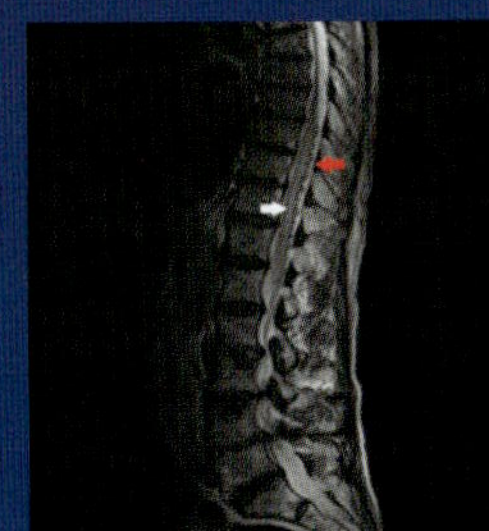

Typical characteristics of a spinal dural arteriovenous fistula (SDAVF) on magnetic resonance imaging (MRI), as represented by the case herein reported. Images of the T2-weighted sequence: centromedullary edema represented by spinal cord hyperintensity (*white arrow*) and dilated posterior veins shown as serpiginous flow voids (*red arrow*)

Nitin Agarwal
David T. Fernandes Cabral
Regan Shanahan

Thieme

Spinal Dural Arteriovenous Fistula-Part III

SDAVFs are often associated with insidious onset and progressive neurological deficits, and the thoracolumbar region (T12–L2) is the most common site of involvement

MANAGEMENT

Endovascular Embolization

- Embolization of the feeding artery (typically radicular artery) using coils or liquid embolic agents
- High success rate (>90%) when performed early
- Postembolization: Close monitoring for potential complications such as spinal cord ischemia or hemorrhage
- Postprocedure, patients may experience gradual improvement in symptoms, although full recovery is rare

Resection

- Indications: Reserved for inaccessible lesions (e.g., those that cannot be reached via the arterial system) or in the cases where endovascular embolization fails
- Surgical approach: Can involve laminectomy for direct access to the fistula or spinal cord decompression
- Outcome: Success largely depends on the timing of intervention and the extent of preexisting spinal cord damage

Prognosis

- Follow-up imaging is required to ensure complete obliteration of the fistula and to monitor for recurrence (repeat angiography may be necessary)
- Prognosis depends on the duration and severity of symptoms at the time of treatment. Early treatment generally leads to better outcomes, but chronic, untreated SDAVF can result in irreversible spinal cord damage, leaving patients with persistent myelopathy

Nitin Agarwal
David T. Fernandes Cabral
Regan Shanahan

Thieme

Spinal Eosinophilic Granulomas

<1%
of all spinal tumors

Genetic risk
BRAF* and *RAS

Benign histiocytic lesions that may occur in isolation or as a part of Hand–Schuller–Christian disease or Letterer–Siwe disease

PRESENTATION

- Langerhans cell histiocytosis is a rare, clonal proliferative disease of epidermal Langerhans cells
- Localized disease, known as eosinophilic granuloma, most commonly affects the cervical spine and typically occurs within the first two decades of life
- Signs and symptoms of spinal cord or nerve root compression include localized back or neck pain, radicular pain, sensory and motor deficits, bladder and bowel dysfunction, and gait disturbances

RADIOGRAPHIC FEATURES

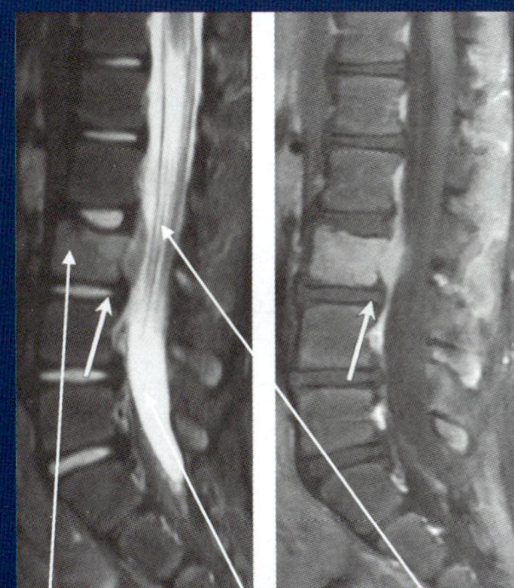

T2 and T1 MRI of an eosinophilic granuloma (white arrow) involving the L3 vertebral body. The lesion extends posteriorly into the epidural space

TREATMENT

- Diagnosis of Langerhans cell histiocytosis requires histological examination, confirmed by CD1a and S-100 staining
- Treatment for Langerhans cell histiocytosis associated with systemic conditions, such as Hand–Schüller–Christian and Letterer–Siwe disease, often involves biopsy and immobilization
- Cases with vertebral collapse or neurological deficits may require decompression and/or spinal fusion
- Low-dose radiotherapy may also be an effective therapy

Further Reading
1. Hassan BW, Moon BJ, Kim YJ, Kim SD, Choi KY, Lee JK. Langerhans cell histiocytosis in the adult lumbar spine: case report. Springerplus 2016;5(1):1398
2. Greenberg MS. Greenberg's Handbook of Neurosurgery. 10th ed. Stuttgart, Germany: Thieme Medical Publishing Group; 2023

Nitin Agarwal
David T. Fernandes Cabral
Samuel Adida

Thieme

Spinal Hemangiomas

Estimated to be found in
10–12%
of the general population

- **Spinal hemangiomas are often discovered incidentally, and biopsy is not needed for diagnosis**
- **Observation for asymptomatic lesions is appropriate**
- **Vertebroplasty or kyphoplasty may be utilized for hemangiomas presenting with pain**
- **Decompressive surgery may be indicated for hemangiomas presenting with deficits or intractable pain**

ETIOLOGY

- Spinal hemangiomas are benign vascular tumors involving the proliferation of capillary and venous structures
- They are the most common primary tumors of the spine located primarily in the lower thoracic and lumbar region

PRESENTATION

- Most spinal hemangiomas are incidental and asymptomatic, with roughly 1% being symptomatic
- May present with pain localized to the level of involvement without radiculopathy. Pain is more often due to compression fractures, herniated discs, or spinal stenosis than the tumor itself

RADIOGRAPHIC FEATURES

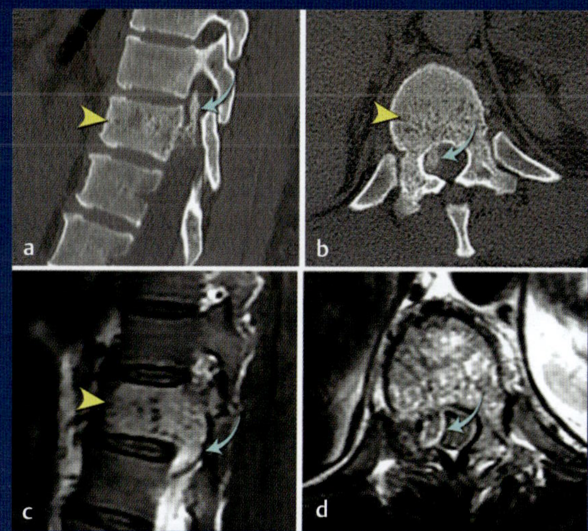

CT and MRI of a vertebral hemangioma in the thoracic spine. Note the proliferation of the hemangioma in the vertebral body (yellow arrows) and extension into the spinal cord (blue arrows)

TREATMENT

- Asymptomatic hemangiomas are treated with routine follow-up. Biopsy may be indicated with atypical features on imaging
- Embolization can be used alone or as a surgical adjunct to reduce operative blood loss
- Surgery is the primary treatment for vertebral hemangiomas producing severe or rapidly progressive neurological deficits, or in lesions that fail to respond to conservative management
- Intralesional resection results in a low recurrence rate (3%). With subtotal resection, the recurrence rate is 20–30% at 2 years

Further Reading

1. Tafti D, Cecava ND. Spinal Hemangioma. StatPearls. Treasure Island, FL: StatPearls Publishing; 2023
2. Teferi N, Abukhiran I, Noeller J et al. Vertebral hemangiomas: diagnosis and management. A single center experience. Clin Neurol Neurosurg 2020;190:105745
3. Patel S, Ansari D, Patil SN et al. High-grade spinal hemangioma: a national cancer database analysis. World Neurosurg 2021;148:e527–e535
4. Greenberg MS. Greenberg's Handbook of Neurosurgery. 10th ed. Stuttgart, Germany: Thieme Medical Publishing Group; 2023

Nitin Agarwal
David T. Fernandes Cabral
Samuel Adida

Thieme

Spine Infection-Part I

MRI with contrast is the gold standard for diagnosing spinal infections, distinguishing between osteomyelitis, diskitis, and epidural abscess

CLINICAL OVERVIEW

Introduction

- Spinal infections encompass a spectrum of pyogenic, granulomatous, and postoperative infections, often leading to vertebral destruction, epidural abscess formation, and neurological compromise. Early recognition and intervention are critical to prevent permanent deficits and sepsis

Classification

- Vertebral osteomyelitis (VO):
    - Infection of the vertebral body, typically via hematogenous spread (e.g., endocarditis, IV drug use)
    - Most common organism: *Staphylococcus aureus* (~50–60%)
    - Other causes: *Escherichia coli* (UTI source), *Pseudomonas* (IVDU), *Brucella* (endemic regions), *Mycobacterium tuberculosis* (Pott's disease)
    - Progresses to bony destruction, disk collapse, and deformity
- Diskitis:
    - Direct infection of the intervertebral disk, usually seen in pediatric patients (vascularized disk) or secondary to VO in adults
    - Can be a precursor to epidural abscess formation
- Spinal epidural abscess:
    - Purulent collection in the epidural space, causing spinal cord/cauda equina compression
    - Triad: Back pain, fever, progressive neurological deficits
    - Rapid deterioration (spinal cord compression) = neurosurgical emergency
- Spinal subdural and intramedullary abscess:
    - Rare, but devastating infections of the subdural space or spinal cord parenchyma, requiring urgent drainage

Nitin Agarwal
David T. Fernandes Cabral
Regan Shanahan
Thieme

Spine Infection-Part II

Spinal epidural abscess requires urgent intervention if neurological deficits develop, with early surgical decompression improving outcomes

Key risk factors for spinal infections include diabetes, immunosuppression (HIV, steroids, chemotherapy), IV drug use, recent spinal surgery, and chronic infections (e.g., endocarditis, UTIs)

IMAGING AND DIAGNOSIS

- MRI with contrast (gold standard):
  - Osteomyelitis: T1 hypointensity, T2/STIR hyperintensity, enhancement of vertebral body ± disk involvement
  - Diskitis: Loss of disk height, enhancement, adjacent marrow edema
  - Epidural abscess: Rim-enhancing fluid collection compressing the thecal sac
- CT-guided biopsy: Essential for culture-directed therapy, especially in nonpyogenic infections (e.g., TB, fungal)
- Blood work: ↑ ESR/CRP (sensitive, but nonspecific):
  - Blood cultures positive in ~50–60% of cases (guides empiric therapy)

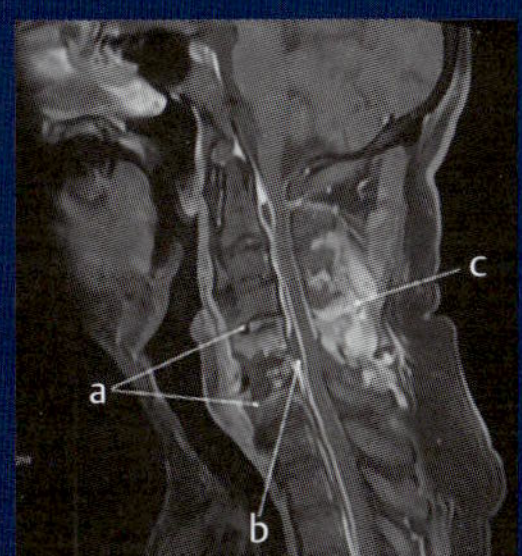

Contrast-enhanced magnetic resonance imaging (CE-MRI) of cervical spine sagittal view. (a) Spondylodiskitis at the C5–C7 level and collapse of C6 vertebral body. (b) Epidural abscess noted at the cervical region extending cranially from C2 below downward. (c) Inflammatory changes involving the paravertebral and paraspinal muscles

MANAGEMENT

Medical Therapy (First-line Therapy for Most Cases)
- Empiric IV antibiotics (6–12 weeks): Cover *S. aureus*, gram-negatives, and anaerobes until culture results
- Antibiotic selection based on biopsy and blood cultures
- TB infections: Prolonged multidrug regimen (rifampin based)

Surgical Intervention
- Indications:
  - Neurological deficits (epidural abscess, spinal cord compression)
  - Progressive deformity/instability (vertebral destruction, kyphosis)
  - Failure of medical therapy or sepsis
- Surgical options:
  - Laminectomy and drainage (abscess)
  - Anterior corpectomy and reconstruction (severe VO with instability)

Nitin Agarwal
David T. Fernandes Cabral
Regan Shanahan

Thieme

Spondylosis-Part I

Cervical spondylosis is the most common cause of myelopathy in adults over 55

Anterior cervical diskectomy and fusion (ACDF) is the most commonly performed surgery for cervical spondylosis with radiculopathy or myelopathy, providing decompression and stabilization

OVERVIEW

- Spondylosis refers to the chronic degenerative changes affecting the spine, encompassing the vertebral bodies, intervertebral disks, facet joints, and surrounding ligaments
- These changes are part of the natural aging process but may be accelerated by mechanical stress, trauma, or genetic predisposition

Pathophysiology of spondylosis:

- Degenerative disk disease (DDD): Loss of disk hydration due to decreased proteoglycan content results in reduced disk height and elasticity
    - Disk collapse increases load on the facet joints and vertebral bodies, accelerating degenerative changes
- Osteophyte formation: Bony projections form along the margins of vertebral bodies and facet joints as a response to chronic stress
- Facet joint arthritis: Degenerative changes in the facet joints, including cartilage erosion and subchondral bone remodeling, contribute to pain and stiffness
    - Facet hypertrophy can further narrow the neural foramina
- Ligamentous hypertrophy and calcification: The ligamentum flavum and other spinal ligaments may thicken and calcify, contributing to spinal canal narrowing and stenosis
- Spinal instability: Progressive degeneration can lead to segmental instability or deformity, such as spondylolisthesis, especially in the lumbar spine

CLINICAL FEATURES

General symptoms:

- Pain: Localized to the affected region (neck, mid-back, or lower back) and may radiate if there is nerve involvement
- Stiffness: Reduced range of motion, especially after periods of inactivity or prolonged use
- Neurological symptoms: Depending on the severity, patients may present with radiculopathy, myelopathy, or neurogenic claudication

Cervical spondylosis: Neck pain and stiffness, often radiating to the shoulders or arms

- Cervical radiculopathy: Pain, numbness, and weakness along the dermatomes of affected nerve roots
- Cervical myelopathy: Gait instability, clumsiness, hyperreflexia, and bowel/bladder dysfunction due to spinal cord compression

Thoracic spondylosis:

- Less common due to the relative immobility of the thoracic spine.
- May present with mid-back pain or, in severe cases, spinal cord compression causing lower extremity weakness or sensory changes

Lumbar spondylosis: Low back pain, often exacerbated by activity or prolonged sitting

- Lumbar radiculopathy (sciatica): Sharp, radiating pain, numbness, or weakness in the legs due to nerve root compression
- Neurogenic claudication: Pain, weakness, or paresthesia in the legs exacerbated by walking and relieved by sitting, commonly seen in lumbar stenosis

Nitin Agarwal
David T. Fernandes Cabral
Samuel Adida

Thieme

Spondylosis-Part II

Lumbar spondylosis can result in neurogenic claudication or radiculopathy due to canal or foraminal narrowing and is managed with lumbar fusion

MANAGEMENT

Neurological examination:
- Motor strength and sensation
- Reflexes: Hyperreflexia may indicate spinal cord compression, while hyporeflexia suggests nerve root compression
- Spurling's test (cervical spine): Reproduction of radicular symptoms with neck extension and lateral bending indicates nerve root compression
- Straight leg raise (lumbar spine): Positive test suggests lumbar radiculopathy
- Gait analysis: Evaluate for ataxia or spastic gait in cases of myelopathy

Imaging studies:
- X-ray: Demonstrates loss of disk height, osteophytes, facet hypertrophy, and spinal alignment abnormalities
- MRI: Gold standard for visualizing soft tissue structures, including intervertebral disks, spinal cord, and nerve roots
- CT: Useful for assessing bony anatomy, including osteophytes and facet joint degeneration
- Electrodiagnostic studies: EMG and nerve conduction studies can differentiate radiculopathy from peripheral neuropathy

Treatment of spondylosis
- Medications: NSAIDs for pain and inflammation, muscle relaxants for spasm, neuropathic agents (e.g., gabapentin) for radiculopathy
- Physical therapy:
- Injections: Epidural steroid injections for radicular pain; facet joint injections or medial branch blocks for facet-mediated pain
- Lifestyle modifications: Weight loss, ergonomic adjustments, and regular exercise

Surgical management (indications):
- Persistent pain despite conservative therapy
- Progressive neurological deficits (e.g., myelopathy or radiculopathy)
- Severe spinal stenosis or deformity
- Common surgical procedures:
- Cervical spine:
  - ACDF: Most common for cervical radiculopathy or myelopathy
  - Laminoplasty or laminectomy: For multilevel spinal stenosis or myelopathy
- Lumbar spine:
  - Laminectomy: Decompression for lumbar spinal stenosis
  - Diskectomy: Removal of herniated disks causing radiculopathy
  - Fusion: For instability or spondylolisthesis

Nitin Agarwal
David T. Fernandes Cabral
Samuel Adida

Thieme

Thoracic Spine-Part I

Thoracic spine pathology commonly affects the thoracolumbar junction (T11–L2) because it bears transitional biomechanical stress, making it prone to fractures and metastatic disease

The thoracic spine's natural kyphosis provides stability but, when exaggerated (e.g., Scheuermann's disease, fractures), can lead to significant pain, pulmonary compromise, and spinal cord compression requiring surgical intervention

ANATOMY

- Vertebral bodies: Larger than cervical vertebrae, with a heart-shaped body. Increase in size from T1 to T12 to support greater weight
- Spinous processes: Long, downward-sloping spinous processes that overlap, especially in the mid-thoracic region
- Costal facets: Present on vertebral bodies and transverse processes, articulating with ribs to form costovertebral and costotransverse joints
- Spinal canal: Narrower than in cervical and lumbar regions, increasing the risk of spinal cord compression in pathology

Biomechanics:

- Mobility: The thoracic spine has limited flexion, extension, and lateral bending due to the ribcage and overlapping spinous processes
    - Rotation is the primary motion, especially in the upper thoracic levels
- Kyphotic curve: The natural kyphosis of the thoracic spine plays a role in overall spinal alignment and load distribution

PHYSICAL EXAMINATION

1. Inspection: Observe for spinal curvature or deformities (e.g., kyphosis, scoliosis); look for asymmetry in the ribcage, muscle atrophy, or visible masses
2. Palpation:
    - Palpate the spinous processes of T1–T12 for tenderness, step-offs, or deformities (e.g., fractures or metastatic lesions)
    - Assess paraspinal muscles for spasm, swelling, or pain
    - Palpate the costovertebral joints for tenderness, which may indicate rib dysfunction or inflammation
3. Range of motion (ROM): Flexion, extension, lateral bend, rotation
4. Neurological testing:

- Dermatomes:
    - T4: Nipple line.
    - T6: Xiphoid process.
    - T10: Umbilicus.
- Motor testing:
    - Evaluate intercostal muscles indirectly by observing breathing mechanics; weakness may indicate thoracic nerve root involvement

5. Special tests:
    - Adam's forward bend test: Assess for scoliosis by observing asymmetry of the ribcage when the patient bends forward
    - Percussion test: Gently percuss over the spinous processes to check for pain, often indicative of fractures or infection
    - Chest expansion test: Reduced chest wall expansion may suggest ankylosing spondylitis or other restrictive pathology

Nitin Agarwal
David T. Fernandes Cabral
Samuel Adida

Thieme

Thoracic Spine-Part II

Although uncommon, thoracic disk herniations are more likely to cause spinal cord compression due to the narrow canal. Symptoms often include thoracic myelopathy, radicular pain, or band-like chest pain

PATHOLOGY & MANAGEMENT

Pathology:
- Compression fractures: Often due to osteoporosis or trauma, particularly at T11–L2
- Thoracic disk herniation: Rare but more likely to cause spinal cord compression due to the narrow canal
- Kyphotic deformities: Scheuermann's kyphosis, postural kyphosis, or secondary to fractures
- Spinal cord compression: Often due to metastases, disk herniation, or epidural abscesses

Thoracic decompression surgery:
- Indications: Spinal cord or nerve root compression due to herniated disks, fractures, metastases, or epidural abscesses
- Procedure: A laminectomy or costotransversectomy is performed to decompress the spinal cord and nerve roots
    - May involve removal of a disk or tumor

Thoracic spinal fusion:
- Indications: Instability or deformity (e.g., fractures, scoliosis, kyphosis)
- Procedure: Hardware (pedicle screws and rods) is used to stabilize the spine
    - Bone grafts are placed to promote fusion
    - May be performed via posterior, anterior, or lateral (thoracoscopic) approaches

Vertebroplasty and kyphoplasty:
- Indications: Painful compression fractures, often due to osteoporosis
- Procedure: Vertebroplasty involves injecting cement into the fractured vertebra
    - Kyphoplasty uses a balloon to restore vertebral height before cement injection

Nitin Agarwal
David T. Fernandes Cabral
Samuel Adida

Thieme

Peripheral Nerves

Axillary Nerve Injury-Part I

Axillary nerve is most commonly injured in anterior shoulder dislocations; always assess for deltoid weakness and lateral shoulder numbness in trauma cases

ANATOMY

- Origin: Posterior cord of the brachial plexus (C5–C6)
- Pathway:
    - Passes posteriorly through the quadrilateral space, along with the posterior circumflex humeral artery
    - Innervates the deltoid and teres minor muscles
    - Gives off the superolateral brachial cutaneous nerve, providing sensation over the lateral shoulder
- Motor:
    - Deltoid: Shoulder abduction (especially past 15 degrees)
    - Teres minor: External rotation and stabilization of the shoulder
- Sensory: Regimental badge area (lateral upper arm)

Symptoms
- Impaired abduction beyond 15 degrees due to deltoid paralysis (supraspinatus initiates abduction)
- Weakness in external rotation (teres minor involvement, though infraspinatus primarily controls this)
- Sensory deficit: Numbness or paresthesia over the regimental badge area (lateral upper arm)
- Muscle atrophy: Visible deltoid wasting in chronic cases

Further Reading

1. Janis JE. Essentials of Plastic Surgery. 3rd ed. New York, NY: Thieme; 2022

Nitin Agarwal
David T. Fernandes Cabral
Samuel Adida

Thieme

Axillary Nerve Injury-Part II

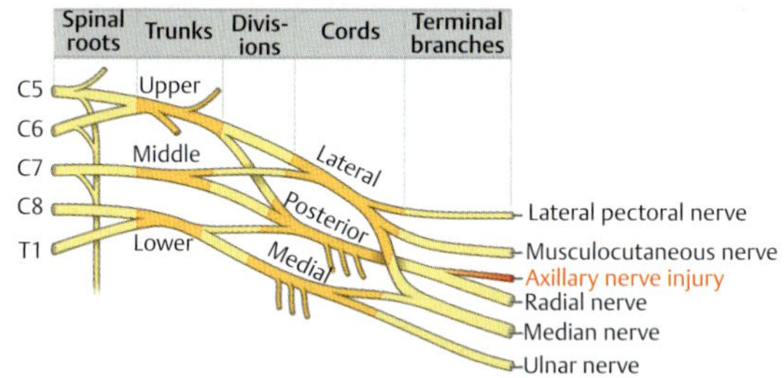

ETIOLOGY & EXAMINATION

Examination

- Weak shoulder abduction (past 15 degrees): Initiation (0–15 degrees) is preserved (supraspinatus–suprascapular nerve)
- Deltoid paralysis causes significant weakness past this range
- Weak external rotation: If teres minor is involved, external rotation is affected (though infraspinatus can compensate)
- Sensation testing: Loss of sensation over the lateral upper arm confirms sensory involvement
- Quadrilateral space syndrome tests: Symptoms worsen with shoulder abduction and external rotation (due to nerve compression)

Etiology

- Trauma:
  - Anterior shoulder dislocation (most common cause)
  - Proximal humeral fractures, especially at the surgical neck
  - Direct blunt trauma to the shoulder
- Iatrogenic injury:
  - Shoulder surgery: Total shoulder arthroplasty, rotator cuff repair, or humeral fixation
  - Improper intramuscular injections in the deltoid region
- Quadrilateral space syndrome:
  - Compression of the axillary nerve and posterior circumflex humeral artery within the quadrilateral space due to fibrous bands, hypertrophy, or mass lesions
  - Common in overhead athletes (e.g., baseball pitchers)

Nitin Agarwal
David T. Fernandes Cabral
Samuel Adida

Thieme

Axillary Nerve Injury-Part III

- **Axillary nerve injury: Isolated deltoid and teres minor weakness, with no biceps involvement; lateral shoulder numbness**
- **C5–C6 radiculopathy: Involves additional biceps weakness (musculocutaneous nerve) and sensory extending beyond the deltoid region**

MANAGEMENT

Diagnostic Workup

Electromyography (EMG) and nerve conduction studies (NCS):

- Confirms denervation of the deltoid and teres minor
- Helps differentiate from C5–C6 radiculopathy or brachial plexopathy
- MRI of the shoulder: Identifies muscle atrophy, fatty degeneration, or space-occupying lesions in the quadrilateral space
- Ultrasound: Dynamic assessment for nerve compression and muscle changes

Management

- *Nonsurgical Treatment (First Line for Mild to Moderate Cases)*
- Activity modification: Avoid movements exacerbating symptoms
- Physical therapy: Strengthening of supraspinatus, infraspinatus, and scapular stabilizers to compensate for deltoid weakness Range-of-motion exercises to prevent frozen shoulder
- NSAIDs and corticosteroid injections: Reduce inflammation, especially in quadrilateral space syndrome

Surgical Management

(Indications: Persistent Weakness, Severe Nerve Injury, or Mass Lesions)

- Nerve decompression and neurolysis: Quadrilateral space decompression for nerve entrapment
    - Indicated in cases of chronic compression with persistent pain/weakness
- Nerve grafting or transfer: For severe nerve injury with no recovery at 6–12 months
    - Transfer options: Spinal accessory nerve to axillary nerve
- Tendon transfers: For chronic, irreversible deltoid paralysis
    - Pectoralis major or trapezius transfer can restore shoulder function

Nitin Agarwal
David T. Fernandes Cabral
Samuel Adida

Thieme

Brachial Plexus Injuries

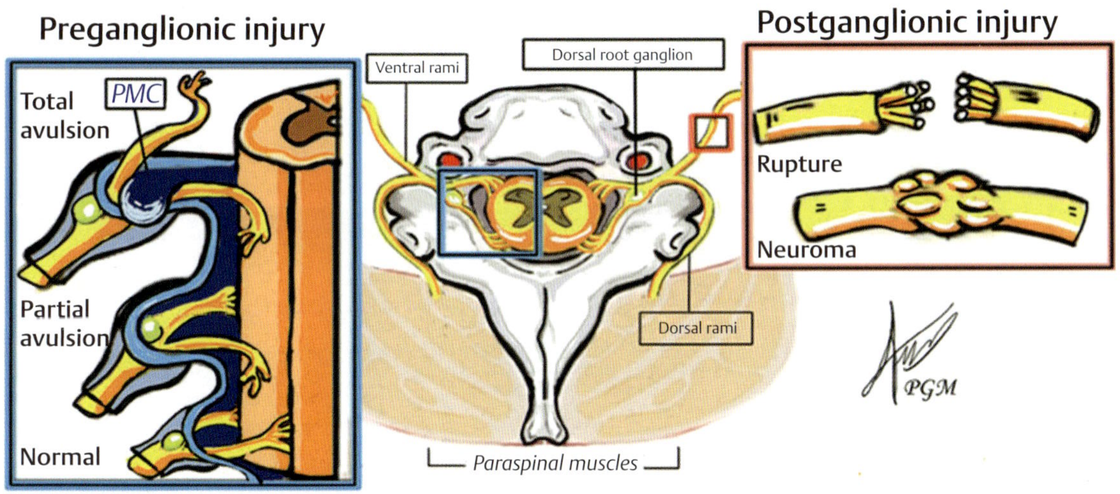

PRESENTATION

- Brachial plexus injuries are caused by neuropraxia, avulsion of nerve roots, or rupture
- Symptoms depend location, chronicity, and mechanism of injury, often including pain, numbness, sensation loss, paresthesias, and weakness or paralysis. Root avulsions may present as muscle paralysis, scapular winging, Horner syndrome, and hemidiaphragm paralysis
- Differential diagnoses are cervical radiculopathy, shoulder joint injury including dislocation or rotator cuff tear, and thoracic outlet syndrome

RADIOGRAPHIC FEATURES

MRI in a 20-year-old male with a brachial plexus injury revealing hyperintense signal suggestive of scarring of the C5 extra-spinal root (solid line) and the upper and middle trunks (dashed line)

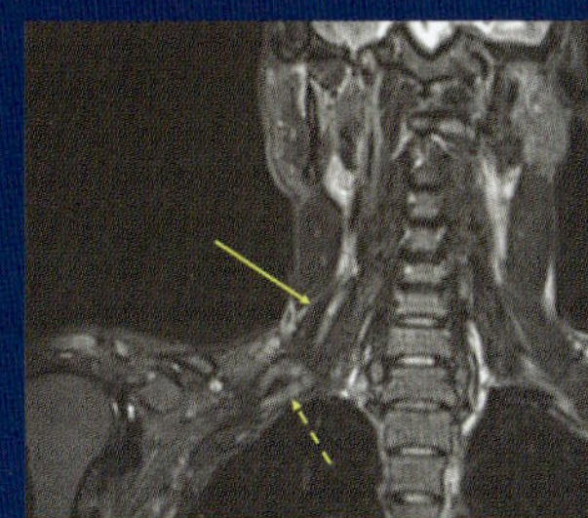

TREATMENT

- There is no chance of spontaneous neural repair with preganglionic injury. Postganglionic injuries including Erb's and Klumpke's palsy at birth are treated conservatively or with surgery
- Surgical management includes neurolysis, nerve grafting, nerve transfer, free functional muscle transfer, and tendon transfer. Dorsal root entry zone (DREZ) lesioning can be performed in patients with intractable pain following avulsion
- Approaches vary depending on upper or lower trunk injury, chronicity, and mechanism of injury

Further Reading

1. Luo TD, Levy ML, Li Z. Brachial Plexus Injuries. In: StatPearls [Internet]. Treasure Island, FL: StatPearls Publishing; 2024
2. Hill JR, Lanier ST, Brogan DM, Dy CJ. Management of adult brachial plexus injuries. J Hand Surg Am 2021;46(9):778–788
3. Greenberg MS. Greenberg's Handbook of Neurosurgery. 10th ed. Stuttgart, Germany: Thieme Medical Publishing Group; 2023

Nitin Agarwal
David T. Fernandes Cabral
Samuel Adida

Thieme

Carpal Tunnel Syndrome

No standard definition exists for the diagnosis, but key indicators include:

- **Being an adult**
- **Paresthesias (with or without pain and numbness) in the median nerve distribution**
- **Nocturnal symptoms**
- **Symptoms worsened or relieved by certain hand or wrist postures or activities**
- **Sparing of the palmar cutaneous branch distribution area**
- **Absence of other clinical explanations**

To aid in diagnosis:

- **EMG and nerve conduction studies are used to help confirm the diagnosis and differentiate it from other pathologies**
- **Wrist MRI and diagnostic ultrasound are the most sensitive**

ETIOLOGY

- Carpal tunnel syndrome is the most common neuropathy in the upper extremity, resulting from compression of the median nerve as it courses through the carpal tunnel
- The age range classically affected by carpal tunnel syndrome is adults aged 40–60 years. Common etiologies include job-related trauma, systemic diseases such as rheumatoid arthritis and diabetes, obesity, pregnancy, and in patients with AV fistulas for hemodialysis

PRESENTATION

- Signs and symptoms include dysesthesias and hypesthesia in the median nerve distribution, hand weakness, decreased grip strength, and clumsiness with fine motor skills
- Phalen's test, Tinel's sign, and ischemic testing can be used to reproduce symptoms

RADIOGRAPHIC FEATURES

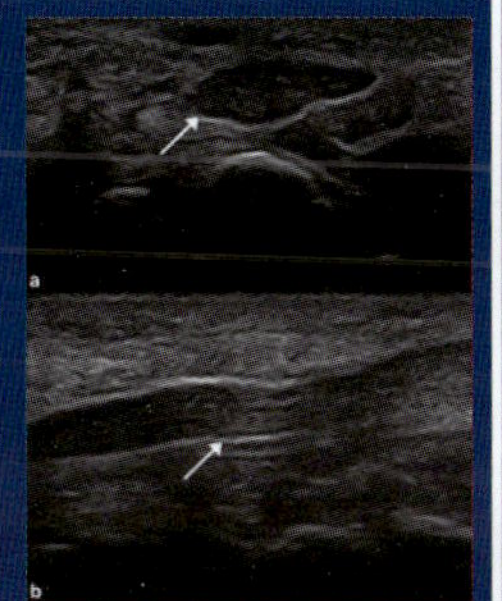

Peripheral nerve high resolution ultrasound image in transverse (a) and longitudinal (b) views of the median nerve at the wrist, showing nerve enlargement at the carpal tunnel

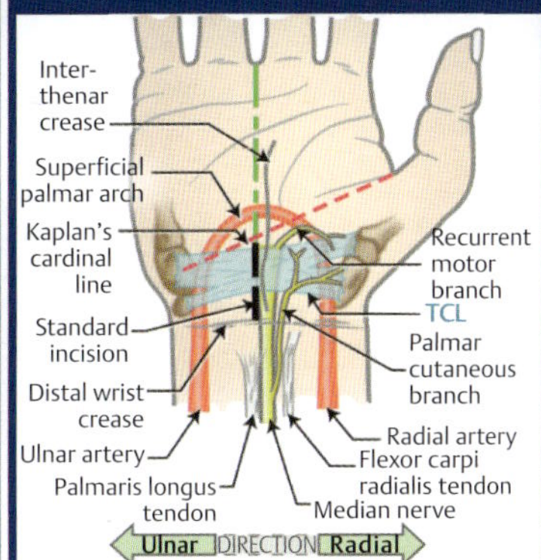

Transpalmar incision for carpal tunnel syndrome (black line). Anatomy can be visualized, including the transverse carpal ligament (blue)

DIFFERENTIAL DIAGNOSES

- Cervical radiculopathy, thoracic outlet syndrome, pronator teres syndrome, de Quervain's syndrome, and tenosynovitis of the flexor ligaments

TREATMENT

- Nonsurgical treatment includes rest, NSAIDs, neutral-position splints, and steroid injections
- Surgical treatment consists of carpal tunnel release via a traditional or transverse incision, or an endoscopic approach, and is indicated for constant numbness, symptoms lasting more than one-year, sensory loss, or thenar weakness or atrophy

Further Reading

1. Dahlin LB, Zimmerman M, Calcagni, M. et al. Carpal tunnel syndrome. Nat Rev Dis Primers 2024;10:37
2. Greenberg MS. Greenberg's Handbook of Neurosurgery. 10th ed. Stuttgart, Germany: Thieme Medical Publishing Group; 2023

Nitin Agarwal
David T. Fernandes Cabral
Samuel Adida

Thieme

Common Peroneal Nerve Entrapment-Part I

Peroneal neuropathy is the most common compressive neuropathy of the lower limb

Onset may be acute, as in trauma episodes (such as in proximal fractures of the fibula), or due to chronic external compressive processes

ANATOMY

The common peroneal nerve, a branch of the sciatic nerve, courses laterally around the fibular neck and bifurcates into the superficial and deep peroneal nerves:

- Superficial peroneal nerve: Innervates the lateral compartment muscles (foot eversion) and supplies sensory innervation to the dorsum of the foot
- Deep peroneal nerve: Innervates the anterior compartment muscles (foot dorsiflexion and toe extension) and provides sensory input to the first web space

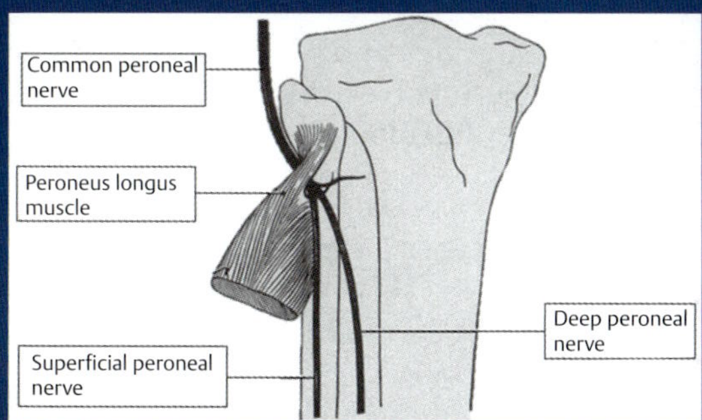

CLINICAL FEATURES

Etiology:
- Compression: Most common cause; typically occurs at the fibular neck due to prolonged leg crossing, squatting, or wearing tight casts/boots
- Trauma: Direct injury to the fibular neck or stretching of the nerve (e.g., knee dislocations, fractures)
- Space-occupying lesions: Ganglion cysts, lipomas, or tumors compressing the nerve
- Systemic conditions: Diabetes mellitus or peripheral neuropathies may predispose to entrapment
- Postsurgical: Iatrogenic injuries during procedures like knee arthroplasty or meniscal repair

Clinical features:
- Motor deficits:
  - Weakness of ankle dorsiflexion (foot drop) due to deep peroneal nerve involvement
  - Weakness of foot eversion due to superficial peroneal nerve involvement
  - L5
- Sensory deficits:
  - Numbness or paresthesia over the dorsum of the foot (superficial peroneal nerve)
  - Loss of sensation in the first web space (deep peroneal nerve)
  - L5
- Tinel's sign: Tingling or pain elicited by tapping over the fibular neck

Nitin Agarwal
David T. Fernandes Cabral
Samuel Adida

Thieme

Common Peroneal Nerve Entrapment-Part II

The main risk factors are related to low body mass index (BMI), or in those who have experienced episodes of rapid weight loss, since they make the nerve more susceptible to compression injuries

PATHOLOGY & MANAGEMENT

Diagnosis:
- Clinical examination: Foot drop and sensory changes are the hallmarks of CPNE
- Electrodiagnostic studies: Nerve conduction studies (NCS) and electromyography (EMG) localize the site of entrapment and assess the degree of nerve injury
- Imaging:
  - MRI: Useful for identifying structural causes such as ganglion cysts or tumors
  - Ultrasound: May reveal nerve thickening or compression and guide interventions

Conservative management:
- Activity modification (avoiding prolonged leg crossing or repetitive knee flexion)
- Ankle-foot orthosis (AFO) for foot drop
- Physical therapy to prevent muscle atrophy and improve gait
- Nonsteroidal anti-inflammatory drugs (NSAIDs) for pain management

Surgical treatment:
- Indications: Persistent symptoms, progressive weakness, or failure of conservative therapy
- Procedure: Nerve decompression via release of constrictive structures around the fibular neck. Removal of compressive lesions (e.g., ganglion cysts) if present
- Postoperative care: Includes physical therapy for motor recovery and prevention of contractures

Prognosis:
- The outcome depends on the severity and duration of nerve compression. Early intervention (conservative or surgical) improves recovery
- Chronic compression or delayed treatment can lead to irreversible axonal damage and persistent deficits

Nitin Agarwal
David T. Fernandes Cabral
Samuel Adida

Thieme

Peripheral Nerve Sheath Tumors-Part I

MRI with contrast is the cornerstone of peripheral nerve tumor evaluation, distinguishing benign, malignant, and infiltrative lesions for surgical planning

OVERVIEW

Introduction

- Peripheral nerve tumors arise from Schwann cells, perineural cells, or fibroblasts, presenting as benign or malignant lesions. While most are benign and slow-growing, malignant transformation, particularly in neurofibromatosis type 1 (NF1), requires early recognition and intervention

Classification

- Benign tumors:
    - Schwannoma: Well encapsulated, eccentric to the nerve, often allowing for enucleation with nerve preservation
    - Neurofibroma: Unencapsulated, infiltrative, often involving multiple fascicles, making nerve-sparing resection challenging
    - Perineurioma: Rare, slow growing, predominantly affecting young adults with progressive neuropathy
- Malignant peripheral nerve sheath tumor (MPNST):
    - Aggressive, locally invasive with a high recurrence rate
    - Strong association with NF1 (>50% of cases)
    - Poor response to chemotherapy and radiation, necessitating radical surgical excision

Nitin Agarwal
David T. Fernandes Cabral
Regan Shanahan

Thieme

Peripheral Nerve Sheath Tumors-Part II

Schwannomas are typically resectable with nerve preservation, while neurofibromas and MPNSTs often require more complex reconstruction strategies due to their infiltrative nature

CLINICAL APPROACH

Clinical Red Flags
- Progressive pain, rapid enlargement, neurological deficits → high suspicion for malignancy
- Tinel's sign: Positive in compressive tumors, though nonspecific

Diagnostic Workup
- MRI with contrast: Gold standard for tumor localization, involvement, and malignancy risk stratification (heterogeneity, necrosis, invasion)
    - Fusiform or round mass with tapered ends
    - Tail sign: Direct communication to a nerve into and/or out of the mass
    - Split fat sign
    - Target sign
    - Iso- or hypointense in the signal related to the skeletal muscle in T1-weighted images, and with increased signal intensity and slightly heterogeneous in T2-weighted images
- On ultrasonography (USG), most PNSTs, including schwannomas, are hypoechogenic and have posterior acoustic reinforcement
- On computed tomography (CT), the typical Schwannoma is characterized as an oval-shaped lesion with soft tissue density, heterogeneous, generally with well-defined limits, established by the encapsulation, and they may also present cystic degeneration
- Electrophysiology (EMG/NCS): Useful for functional assessment but limited in differentiating tumor types
- Biopsy: Reserved for suspected malignancies or unresectable tumors due to the risk of iatrogenic nerve injury

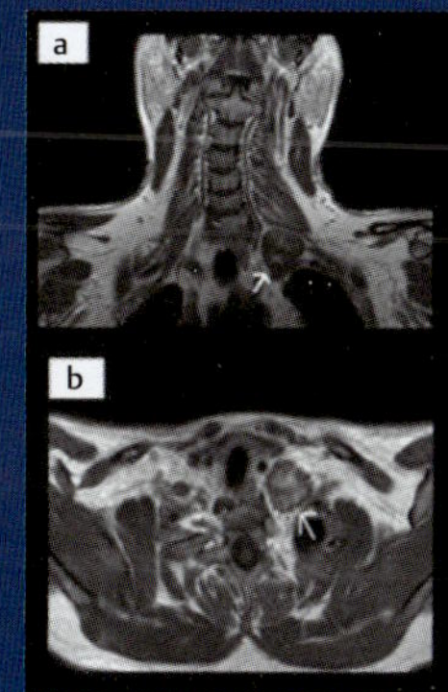

Magnetic resonance imaging with and without contrast of the brachial plexus demonstrated a 4- to 6-cm homogeneously enhancing lesion (*white arrow*) on (a) T1-weighted coronal and (b) axial images. The lesion appeared to arise from the C7 nerve root at the middle trunk of the brachial plexus. Imaging was consistent with a benign peripheral nerve sheath tumor, and pathology confirmed it to be a neurofibroma

Nitin Agarwal
David T. Fernandes Cabral
Regan Shanahan

Thieme

Peripheral Nerve Sheath Tumors-Part III

Rapidly growing or painful nerve tumors in NF1 patients should be presumed malignant until proven otherwise, necessitating early multidisciplinary intervention

MANAGEMENT

- Benign tumors: Observation versus surgical resection based on symptom burden and progression
- Surgical resection:
    - Schwannomas: Enucleation with nerve preservation
    - Neurofibromas: Require fascicular dissection, often with nerve sacrifice in plexiform variants
    - MPNST: Wide-margin resection; adjuvant therapy with limited efficacy

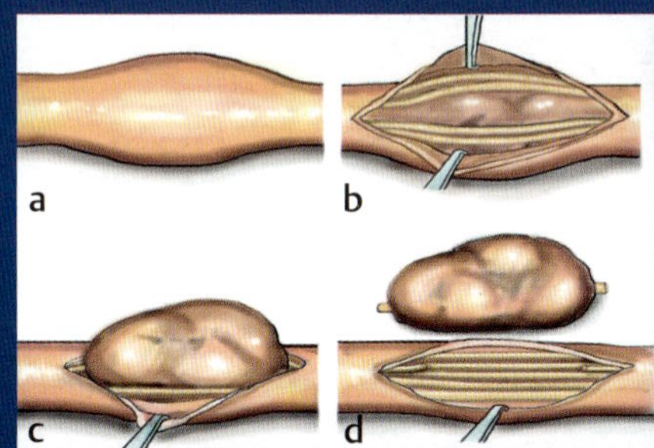

(a) Schwannoma causing bulging in the peripheral nerve. (b) After the opening of the epineurium, it is possible to identify the presence of the tumor involved by viable nervous fascicles. (c) After the correct dissection of the tumor, the fascicles were removed peripherally to preserve them. (d) Complete excision of the Schwannoma is noted with sacrifice only of the bundle that originated it

Nitin Agarwal
David T. Fernandes Cabral
Regan Shanahan

Thieme

Radial Nerve Entrapment

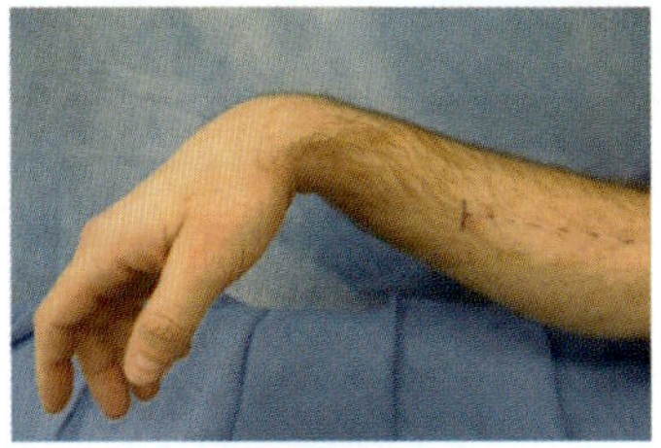

Wrist drop

The posterior interosseous nerve at the level of the proximal forearm is the most common site for radial nerve entrapment

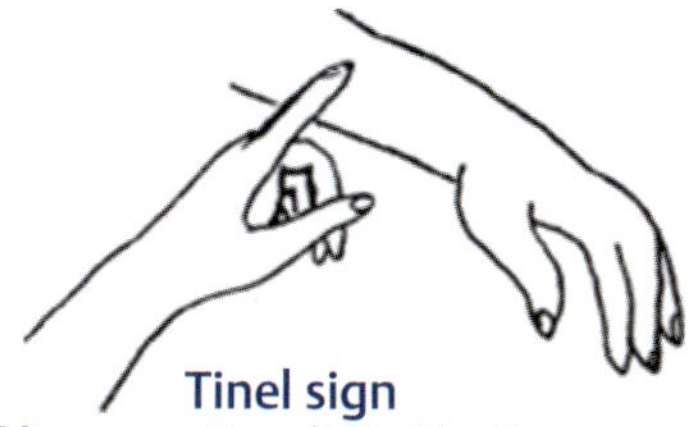

Tinel sign

Tingling or prickling sensation elicited by the percussion of an injured nerve trunk at or distal to the site of the lesion

OVERVIEW

- Radial nerve basic
  - Origin: Posterior cord of the brachial plexus
  - Course: Posteromedially with the axillary vessels, behind the humerus, then anteriorly towards the elbow where it divides into superficial and deep branches
  - Terminal branches: Posterior interosseous (deep) and superficial radial nerves
  - Motor: Elbow, wrist, and finger extension
  - Sensory: Dorsal aspect of the thumb, index and middle fingers
- Work Up
  - Physical exam
  - Imaging
    - X-ray (for trauma)
    - MRI (for compressive neuropathies)
    - EMG/NCS
    - Ultrasound

COMPRESSION SYNDROMES

Loss of extension of the forearm, hand, and fingers; sensory loss in the lateral arm and posterior forearm, radiating to the radial aspect of the hand

- Axillary compression
  - Crutch misuse
- Mid-upper arm compression
  - "Saturday night palsy : improper positioning of the arm in sleep
  - Positioning during general anesthesia
  - Callus due to old humeral fracture

Pain in the forearm and wrist, along with weakness with finger metacarpal extension and wrist extension

- Forearm compression
  - Posterior interossesous neuropathy (PIN)
  - Lipomas, ganglia, fibromas, rheumatoid arthritis changes at the elbow, entrapment at the arcade of Frohse
  - Radial tunnel syndrome
    - AKA "Supinator Syndrome"
    - Repeated forceful supination or protonation or inflammation of supinator muscle

COMPRESSION SYNDROMES

Numbness and tingling in the radial half of the dorsum of the hand and the dorsum of the radial 3½ digits, no motor deficits.

- Injury at the level of the forearm
  - Wartenberg syndrome
    - Wearing tight jewelry/watches

TREATMENT

- Treatment
  - NSAIDs
  - Immobilization
  - Physical therapy
  - Corticosteroid injections
  - Surgery (rare)
- Prognosis
  - Up to 92% resolve with observation alone after 3–4 months
  - Most demyelinating injuries fully resolve after one month

Further Reading

1. Tsementzis S ed. Trigeminal neuralgia. In: Differential Diagnosis in Neurology and Neurosurgery: A clinician's Pocket Guide. 2nd ed. Noida: Thieme; 2022
2. Gagliardi F, Gragnaniello C, Mortini P et al. eds. Intradural exposure. In: Operative Cranial Neurosurgical Anatomy 1st ed. Noida: Thieme; 2018

Nitin Agarwal
David T. Fernandes Cabral
Samuel Adida

Thieme

Suprascapular Nerve Injury-Part I

C5–C6 radiculopathy presents with similar weakness but involves deltoid involvement (axillary nerve) and sensory changes, which SSN injury does not

ANATOMY

- Origin: Upper trunk of the brachial plexus (C5–C6)
- Pathway: Passes through the suprascapular notch, beneath the transverse scapular ligament
- Supplies the supraspinatus muscle in the supraspinous fossa
- Travels around the spinoglenoid notch, supplying the infraspinatus muscle in the infraspinous fossa
- Function:
  - Motor: Supraspinatus (initiates abduction) and infraspinatus (external rotation)
  - Sensory: Small contribution to the acromioclavicular and glenohumeral joints

Symptoms:
- Dull, aching posterior shoulder pain, often radiating to the lateral arm
- Weakness:
  - Suprascapular notch compression: Weakness in shoulder abduction (supraspinatus) and external rotation (infraspinatus)
  - Spinoglenoid notch compression: Isolated external rotation weakness (infraspinatus)
- Muscle atrophy:
  - Visible wasting of the supraspinatus and infraspinatus muscles in chronic cases

Differential diagnosis:
- Pathology around the shoulder joint
- Parsonage–Turner: Limited to the suprascapular nerve
- Cervical radiculopathy
- Upper brachial plexus lesion

Nitin Agarwal
David T. Fernandes Cabral
Samuel Adida

Thieme

Suprascapular Nerve Injury-Part II

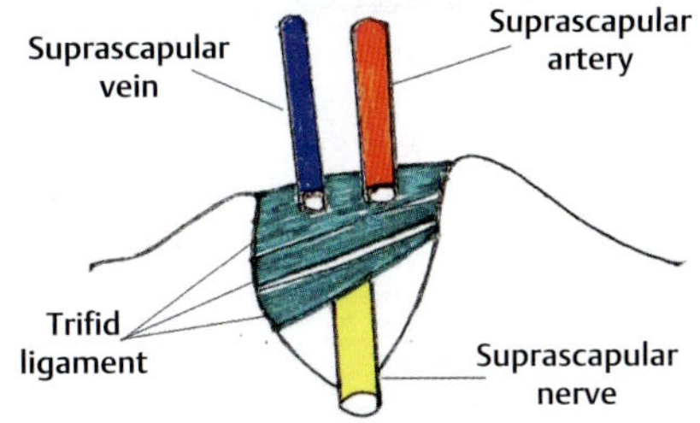

ETIOLOGY & EXAMINATION

Examination:
- Weak shoulder abduction (first 15 degrees): Suggests supraspinatus involvement
- Weak external rotation: Suggests infraspinatus involvement
- Palpation of the suprascapular notch: May elicit tenderness if entrapment is present
- Cross-body adduction test: Can worsen symptoms due to nerve traction
- Hornblower's sign: Severe weakness of external rotation in infraspinatus paralysis

Etiology:
- Entrapment neuropathy:
  - Suprascapular notch entrapment: Affects both the supraspinatus and infraspinatus
  - Spinoglenoid notch entrapment: Affects only the infraspinatus (external rotation weakness without abduction deficits); spares supraspinatus function and presents primarily with external rotation weakness
- Trauma:
  - Fractures of the scapula, clavicle, or humerus
  - Shoulder dislocations (especially posterior dislocations)
- Repetitive overhead activities:
  - Common in athletes (e.g., baseball pitchers, volleyball players) and manual laborers
- Mass lesions:
  - Ganglion cysts (often associated with labral tears)
  - Tumors compressing the nerve at the suprascapular or spinoglenoid notch

Nitin Agarwal
David T. Fernandes Cabral
Samuel Adida

Thieme

Suprascapular Nerve Injury-Part III

Entrapment at the suprascapular notch affects both the supraspinatus and infraspinatus muscles. Transverse scapular ligament release or spinoglenoid notch decompression can significantly improve function in refractory cases

MANAGEMENT

Diagnostic workup:
Electromyography (EMG) and nerve conduction studies (NCS):
- Confirms denervation of the supraspinatus and/or infraspinatus
- Helps differentiate from cervical radiculopathy (C5–C6)

MRI of the shoulder: Identifies muscle atrophy, fatty degeneration, and compressive lesions (e.g., ganglion cysts).
Ultrasound: Dynamic assessment for nerve impingement and muscle atrophy

Management:
Nonsurgical treatment (first line for mild to moderate cases):
- Activity modification: Avoid overhead movements
- Physical therapy: Strengthening of rotator cuff and scapular stabilizers, range-of-motion exercises to prevent stiffness
- NSAIDs and corticosteroid injections: Reduce inflammation if associated with impingement

Surgical management
(indications: persistent symptoms, severe weakness, or mass lesions):
- Suprascapular nerve decompression: Release of the transverse scapular ligament at the suprascapular notch
- Spinoglenoid notch decompression if isolated infraspinatus involvement
- Cyst excision: Ganglion cysts at the spinoglenoid notch can be excised to relieve nerve compression
- Shoulder stabilization procedures: If nerve injury is secondary to recurrent shoulder dislocations

Nitin Agarwal
David T. Fernandes Cabral
Samuel Adida

Thieme

Tarsal Tunnel Syndrome

- **Etiology: Caused by compression of the posterior tibial nerve, often due to trauma, systemic diseases such as diabetes mellitus, or deformity like flat foot. 20% of cases are idiopathic**
- **Presentation: Pain, tingling, and burning in the medial ankle and plantar foot, worsened by weight bearing. Physical examinations may show positive Tinel's sign and the dorsiflexion–eversion test**
- **Management: Conservative treatment includes activity modification and NSAIDs. Surgery (flexor retinaculum release) is for severe cases or failure of conservative measures**

To aid in diagnosis:

- **EMG and nerve conduction studies are used to help confirm diagnosis from other pathologies**
- **Foot MRI and diagnostic ultrasound are most sensitive**

PRESENTATION

- Tarsal tunnel syndrome (TTS) is a compressive neuropathy of the posterior tibial nerve and its branches within the tarsal tunnel beneath the flexor retinaculum
- Etiology:
  - Extrinsic causes: Poor footwear, trauma, systemic disease (e.g., diabetes mellitus), and biomechanical deformities (e.g., flat foot)
  - Intrinsic causes: Space-occupying lesions (e.g., ganglion cysts, lipomas), hypertrophic retinaculum, and vascular anomalies
  - 20% of cases are idiopathic
- Presentation:
  - Symptoms: Pain, dysesthesia, paresthesia, burning, or tingling in the medial ankle and plantar foot, worsened by weight bearing and relieved by rest
  - Physical examination: Tinel's sign, dorsiflexion–eversion test, and Valleix phenomenon
- Differential diagnoses include plantar fasciitis, lumbar radiculopathy (L5–S1), Morton's neuroma, peripheral neuropathy, and arthritis

TREATMENT

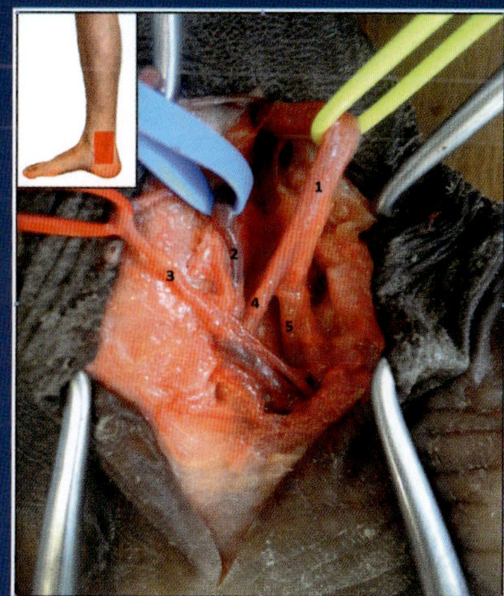

Compression of the tibial nerve at the medial malleolus. The flexor retinaculum is sectioned, revealing the tibial nerve division into medial and lateral plantar nerves. Shown are the tibial nerve (1), posterior tibial vein (2), posterior tibial artery (3), medial plantar nerve (4), and lateral plantar nerve (5)

- Conservative management:
  - Activity modification and PT
  - Pain management: NSAIDs, corticosteroid injections, and TCAs
- Surgical management :
  - Indications: Failed conservative management, clear entrapment cause, or severe symptoms
  - Procedure: Flexor retinaculum release from the medial malleolus to the sustentaculum tali; may be ultrasound guided
  - Predictors of success: Positive Tinel's sign presurgery, early diagnosis, short symptom duration, and no prior ankle pathology
  - Outcomes: Success rates range from 44 to 96%, with better results in younger patients and those with identifiable causes
  - Prognosis: Variable; favorable with early intervention. Poor outcomes when no clear etiology or failed conservative management. Mixed evidence on benefits of surgical decompression in patients with diabetes

Further Readings

1. Rodríguez-Merchán EC, Moracia-Ochagavía I. Tarsal tunnel syndrome: current rationale, indications and results. EFORT Open Rev 202;6(12):1140–1147

Nitin Agarwal
David T. Fernandes Cabral
Samuel Adida

Thieme

Ulnar Nerve Entrapment

- **Sites of compression: Cubital tunnel (elbow) and Guyon's canal (wrist)**
- **Motor and sensory deficits: Ulnar nerve compression affects the intrinsic hand muscles, including the hypothenar eminence, interossei, and the third and fourth lumbricals**
- **Diagnosis and management: Clinical examination (e.g., Froment's and Wartenberg's signs) and imaging. Initial treatment includes NSAIDs, splinting, and PT; surgery may be considered if conservative measures fail, particularly for decompression or nerve transposition**

To aid in diagnosis:

- **EMG and nerve conduction studies are used to help confirm diagnosis from other pathologies**
- **Wrist MRI and diagnostic ultrasound are most sensitive**

PRESENTATION

- Ulnar nerve entrapment commonly occurs at the cubital tunnel (elbow) or Guyon's canal (wrist). Compression leads to motor and sensory deficits in the ulnar nerve distribution distal to compression:
  - Cubital tunnel: Compression typically by Osborne's ligament, affecting motor and sensory function in the forearm and hand
  - Guyon's canal: Compression of the ulnar nerve as it traverses through Guyon's canal
- Symptoms may include numbness, tingling, and weakness in the ulnar distribution (5th finger, ulnar half of the 4th finger, hypothenar eminence). Prolonged compression may cause atrophy and decreased pinch strength (e.g., Froment's sign, Wartenberg's sign)
- Differential diagnoses include cervical radiculopathy (C8–T1), thoracic outlet syndrome, medial epicondylitis, elbow fractures or dislocations, rheumatoid arthritis, Pancoast tumor, and double crush phenomenon (simultaneous nerve compression at two different sites, such as the cervical spine and a peripheral nerve)

RADIOGRAPHIC FEATURES

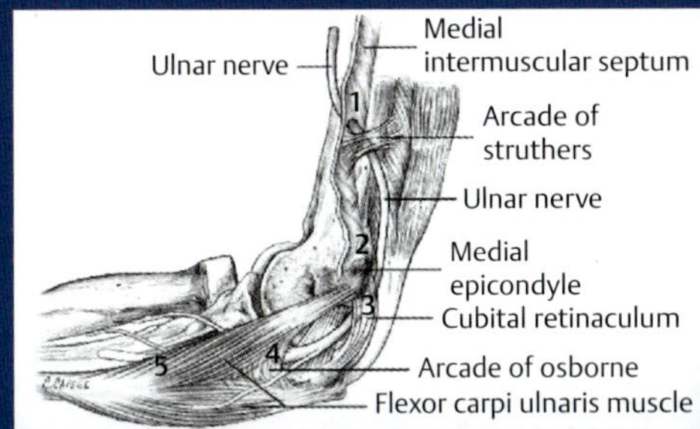

Common sites of ulnar nerve compression including the cubital tunnel

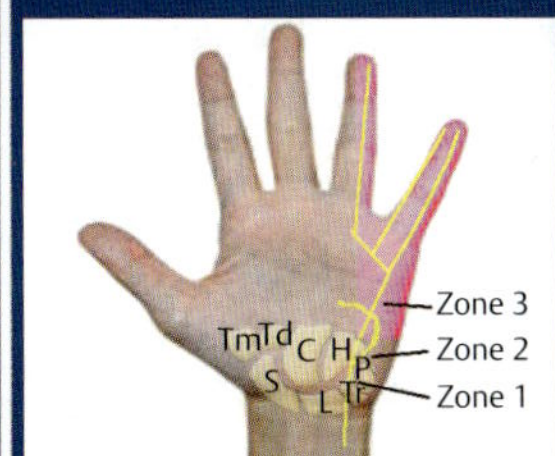

Zones of ulnar nerve compression in Guyon's canal:

- Zone 1: Mixed motor and sensory deficits
- Zone 2: Isolated motor deficits
- Zone 3: Isolated sensory deficits

TREATMENT

- Conservative management :
  - Anti-inflammatory medications (e.g., NSAIDs), padding, physical and occupational therapy for positioning and exercises (e.g., nerve gliding)
  - Lidocaine/steroid injections and splinting (elbow at 45 degrees of flexion, wrist neutral) may improve symptoms for patients avoiding surgery or as a bridge to surgery
- Surgical management:
  - Guyon's canal: Release of compression, or excision of the ganglia or masses causing compression. Zone 2 compression may require release of the pisohamate ligament
  - Cubital tunnel: Ulnar nerve transposition or release of Osborne's ligament
- Prognosis:
  - Conservative management may result in excellent outcomes in mild cases; surgical intervention often leads to near-total symptom relief if compression is adequately addressed

Further Readings

1. Natroshvili T, van de Warenburg MS, Heine EP, Slater NJ, Walbeehm ET, Bartels RHMA. Conservative treatment of ulnar nerve compression at the elbow: a systematic review and meta-analysis. Arch Plast Surg 2023;50(1):70–81
2. Lung BE, Siwiec RM. Anatomy, Shoulder and Upper Limb, Forearm Flexor Carpi Ulnaris Muscle. Treasure Island, FL: StatPearls Publishing; 2025
3. Davis DD, Kane SM. Ulnar Nerve Entrapment. Treasure Island, FL: StatPearls Publishing; 2025

Nitin Agarwal
David T. Fernandes Cabral
Samuel Adida

Thieme